braintrust

braintrust

What Neuroscience Tells Us about Morality

Patricia S. Churchland

Princeton University Press • Princeton and Oxford

It's a vice to trust everyone, and equally a vice to trust no one.

—Seneca

This is our mammalian conflict: what to give to others and what to keep for yourself. Treading that line, keeping others in check and being kept in check by them, is what we call morality.

—Ian McEwan, *Eternal Love*

Contents

Illustrations

braintrust

1. Introduction

Trial by ordeal seemed to me, as I learned about it in school, ridiculously unfair. How could it have endured as an institution in Europe for hundreds of years? The central idea was simple: with God's intervention, innocence would plainly reveal itself, as the accused thief sank to the bottom of the pond, or the accused adulterer remained unburned by the red hot poker placed in his hand. Only the guilty would drown or burn. (For witches, the ordeal was less "forgiving": if the accused witch drowned she was presumed innocent; if she bobbed to the surface, she was guilty, whereupon she was hauled off to a waiting fire.) With time on our hands, my friend and I concocted a plan. She would falsely accuse me of stealing her purse, and then I would lay my hand on the stove and see whether it burned. We fully expected it would burn, and it did. So if the test was that obvious, how could people have trusted to trial by ordeal as a system of justice?

From the medieval clerics, the answer would have been that our test was frivolous, and that God would not deign to intervene with a miracle for the benefit of kids fooling around. That answer seemed to us a bit cooked up. What is the evidence God *ever* intervened on behalf of the wrongly accused? A further difficulty concerned nonbelievers, such as those not yet reached by missionaries, or . . . maybe *me*? Still, this answer alerted us to the matter of metaphysical (or as we said then, "otherworldly") beliefs in moral practices, along with the realization that what seemed to us obvious about fairness in determining guilt might not be obvious after all.

My history teacher tried to put the medieval practice in context, aiming to soften slightly our sense of superiority over our medieval ancestors: in trial by ordeal, the guilty were more likely to confess, since they believed God would not intervene on their behalf, whereas the innocent, convinced that God would help out, were prepared to go to trial. So the system might work pretty well for getting confessions from the guilty, even if it did poorly for protecting the innocent. This answer alerted us to the presence of pragmatics in moral practices, which struck us as a little less lofty than we had been led to expect. How hideously *unfair* if you were innocent and did go to trial. I could visualize myself, bound by ropes, drowning in a river after being accused of witchcraft by my piano teacher.[1]

So what is it to be fair? How do we *know* what to count as fair? Why do we regard trial by ordeal as *wrong*? Thus opens the door into the vast tangled forest of questions about right and wrong, good and evil, virtues and vices. For most of my adult life as a philosopher, I shied away from plunging unreservedly into these sorts of questions about morality. This was largely because I could not see a systematic way through that tangled forest, and because a lot of contemporary moral philosophy, though venerated in academic halls, was completely untethered to the "hard and fast"; that is, it had no strong connection to evolution or to the brain, and hence was in peril of floating on a sea of mere, albeit confident, opinion. And no doubt the medieval clerics were every bit as confident.

It did seem that likely Aristotle, Hume, and Darwin were right: we are social by nature. But what does that actually mean in terms of our *brains* and our *genes*? To make progress beyond the broad hunches about our nature, we need something solid to attach the claim to. Without relevant, real data from evolutionary biology, neuroscience, and genetics, I could not see how to tether ideas about "our nature" to the hard and fast.

Despite being flummoxed, I began to appreciate that recent developments in the biological sciences allow us to see through the tangle, to begin to discern pathways revealed by new data. The phenomenon of moral values, hitherto so puzzling, is now less so. Not entirely clear, just less puzzling. By drawing on converging new data from neuroscience, evolutionary biology, experimental psychology, and genetics, and given a philosophical framework consilient with those data, we can now meaningfully approach the question of where values come from.

The wealth of data can easily swamp us, but the main story line can be set out in a fairly straightforward way. My aim here is to explain what is probably true about our social nature, and what that involves in terms of the neural platform for moral behavior. As will become plain, the platform is *only* the platform; it is not the whole story of human moral values. Social practices, and culture more generally, are not my focus here, although they are, of course, hugely important in the values people live by. Additionally, particular moral dilemmas, such as when a war is a just war, or whether inheritance taxes are fair, are not the focus here.

Although remarks of a general sort concerning our nature often fall on receptive ears, those same ears may become rather deaf when the details of brain circuitry begin to be discussed. When we speak of the possibility of linking large-scale questions about our mind with developments in the neurosciences, there are those who are wont to wag their fingers and warn us about the perils of *scientism*. That means, so far as I can tell, the offense of taking science into places where allegedly it has no business, of being in the grip of the grand delusion that science can explain everything, do everything. Scientism, as I have been duly wagged, is overreaching.

The complaint that a scientific approach to understanding moral-ity commits the sin of scientism does really exaggerate what science is up to, since the scientific enterprise does not aim to displace the arts or the humanities. Shakespeare and Mozart and Caravaggio are not in competition with protein kinases and micro RNA. On the other hand, it is true that philosophical claims about the nature of things, such as moral intuition, are vulnerable. Here, philosophy and science are working the same ground, and evidence should trump armchair reflection. In the present case, the claim is not that science will wade in and tell us for every dilemma what *is* right or wrong. Rather, the point is that a deeper understanding of what it is that makes humans and other animals social, and what it is that disposes us to care about others, may lead to greater understanding of how to cope with social problems. That cannot be a bad thing. As the Scottish philosopher Adam Smith (1723–90) observed, "science is the great antidote to the poison of enthusiasm and superstition." By *enthusiasm* here, he meant *ideological fervor,* and undoubtedly his observation applies especially to the moral domain . Realistically, one must acknowledge in any case that science is not on the brink of explaining everything about the brain or evolution or genetics. We know more now than we did ten years ago; ten years hence we will know even more. But there will always be further questions looming on the horizon.

The scolding may be sharpened, however, warning of the logical absurdity of drawing on the biological sciences to understand the plat-form for morality. Here the accusation is that such an aim rests on the dunce's error of going from an *is* to an *ought*, from *facts* to *values.* Morality, it will be sternly sermonized, tells what we *ought* to do; biol-ogy can only tell what *is* the case.[2] With some impatience, we may be reproached for failing to heed the admonition of another eighteenth-century Scottish philosopher, David Hume (1711–76), that you can-not derive an *ought* statement from statements about what *is.* Hence my project, according to the scold, is muddled and misbegotten. "Stop reading here" would be the advice of the grumbler.

The scold is spurious. First, Hume made his comment in the context of ridiculing the conviction that reason—a simplistic notion of reason as detached from emotions, passions, and cares—is the watershed for morality. Hume, recognizing that basic values are part of our nature, was unwavering: "reason is and ought only to be the slave of the passions."[3] By *passion*, he meant something more general than *emotion*; he had in mind any practical orientation toward performing an action in the social or physical world.[4] Hume believed that moral behavior, though informed by understanding and reflection, is rooted in a deep, widespread, and enduring social motivation, which he referred to as "the moral sentiment." This is part of our biological nature. Hume, like Aristotle before him and Darwin after him, was every inch a naturalist.

So whence the warning about *ought* and *is*? The answer is that precisely because he was a naturalist, Hume had to make it clear that the sophisticated naturalist has no truck with simple, sloppy inferences going from *what is* to *what ought to be*. He challenged those who took moral understanding to be the preserve of the elite, especially the clergy, who tended to make dimwitted inferences between descriptions and prescriptions.[5] For example, it might be said (my examples, not Hume's), "Husbands are stronger than their wives, so wives ought to obey their husbands," or "We have a tradition that little boys work as chimney sweeps, therefore we ought to have little boys work as chimney sweeps," or "It is natural to hate people who are deformed, therefore it is right to hate people who are deformed." These sorts of inferences are stupid, and precisely because Hume was a naturalist, he wanted to dissociate himself from them and their stupidity.

Hume understood that he needed to have a subtle and sensible account of the complex relationship between moral decisions on the one hand, and the dynamic interaction of mental processes—motivations, thoughts, emotions, memories, and plans—on the other. And to a first approximation, he did. He outlined the importance of pain and pleasure in learning social practices and shaping our passions, of institutions and customs in providing a framework for stability and prosperity, of reflection and intelligence in revising existing institutions and customs.[6] He understood that passions and motivations, as well as moral principles, can, and often do, conflict with one another, and that there is individual variability in social temperament.

Thus, to continue in the contemporary idiom, the relation between social urges and the social practices that serve well-being is not simple and certainly not syllogistic; finding good solutions to social problems often requires much wisdom, goodwill, negotiation, historical knowledge, and intelligence. Just as Hume said. Naturalism, while shunning stupid inferences, does nevertheless find the roots of morality in how we are, what we care about, and what matters to us—in our nature. Neither supernaturalism (the otherworldly gods), nor some rarefied, unrealistic concept of reason, explains the moral motherboard.[7]

So how did the idea "you cannot derive an *ought* from an *is*" acquire philosophical standing as the "old reliable" smackdown of a naturalistic approach to morality? First, a semantic clarification helps explain the history. *Deriving* a proposition in deductive logic strictly speaking requires a formally valid argument; that is, the conclusion must deductively follow from the premises, with no leeway, no mere high probability (e.g., "All men are mortal, Socrates is a man, so Socrates is mortal"). Assuming the premises are true, the conclusion must be true. Strictly speaking, therefore, one cannot derive (in the sense of *construct a formally valid argument for*) a statement about what ought to be done from a set of facts about what is the case. The other part of the story is that many moral philosophers, especially those following Kant, thought Hume was just plain wrong in his naturalism, and that biology in general has nothing to teach us about morality per se. So they hung naturalism by the heels on Hume's is/ought observation.

But Hume was right to be a naturalist. In a much broader sense of "infer" than *derive* you can infer (*figure out*) what you ought to do, drawing on knowledge, perception, emotions, and understanding, and balancing considerations against each other. We do it constantly, in both the physical and social worlds. In matters of health, animal husbandry, horticulture, carpentry, education of the young, and a host of other practical domains, we regularly figure out what we ought to do based on the facts of the case, and our background understanding. I have a horrendous toothache? I ought to see a dentist. There is a fire on the stove? I ought to throw baking soda on it. The bear is on my path? I ought to walk quietly, humming to myself, in the orthogonal direction. What gets us around the world is mainly *not* logical deduction (derivation). By and large, our problem-solving operations—the figuring out and the reasoning—look like a *constraint satisfaction* process, not like deduction or the execution of an algorithm. For example, a wolf pack watches the caribou herd, and needs to select a likely victim—an animal that is weak, isolated, or young. The pack is very hungry and needs to be successful, so a lame older animal may be a better choice than a tiny newborn, but it is more risky; the hunters want to conserve energy, but acquire a rich energy source; they need to take into account the location of the river, how they can drive the victim to a waiting pair of wolves, and so forth. Humans encounter similar problems on a regular basis—in buying a car, designing a dwelling, moving to a new job, selecting whether to opt for an aggressive treatment for metastasized cancer, or hospice care. In any case, that most problem-solving is not deduction is clear. Most practical and social problems are constraint satisfaction problems, and our brains often make good decisions in figuring out some solution.[8] What exactly *constraint satisfaction* is in neurobiological terms we do not yet understand, but roughly speaking it involves various factors with various weights and probabilities interacting so as to produce a suitable solution to a question. Not necessarily the best solution, but a suitable solution. The important point for my project, therefore, is straightforward: that you cannot *derive* an *ought* from an *is* has very little bearing so far as in-the-world problem-solving is concerned.

Brains navigate the *causal* world by recognizing and categorizing events they need to care about, given how the animal makes a living—what berries taste good, where juicy termites can be found, how fish can be caught.[9] The hypothesis on offer is that navigation of the *social* world mostly depends on the same neural mechanisms—motivation and drive, reward and prediction, perception and memory, impulse control and decision-making. These same mechanisms can be used to make physical or social decisions; to build world knowledge or social knowledge, such as who is irascible, or when am I expected to share food or defend the group against intruders or back down in a fight.[10]

Social navigation is an instance of causal navigation generally, and shapes itself to the existing ecological conditions. In the social domain, the ecological conditions will include the social behavior of individual group members as well as their cultural practices, some of which get called "moral" or "legal." By and large, humans, like some other highly social mammals, are strongly motivated to be with group members and to share in their practices. Our moral behavior, while more complex than the social behavior of other animals, is similar in that it represents our attempt to manage well in the existing social ecology.

In sum, from the perspective of neuroscience and brain evolution, the routine rejection of scientific approaches to moral behavior based on Hume's warning against deriving *ought* from *is* seems unfortunate, especially as the warning is limited to deductive inferences. The dictum can be set aside for a deeper, albeit programmatic, neurobiological perspective on what reasoning and problem-solving are, how social navigation works, how evaluation is accomplished by nervous systems, and how mammalian brains make decisions.

The truth seems to be that the values rooted in the circuitry for caring—for well-being of self, offspring, mates, kin, and others—shape social reasoning about many issues: conflict resolution, keeping the peace, defense, trade, resource distribution, and many other aspects of social life in all its vast richness. Not only do these values and their material basis constrain social problem-solving, they are at the same time facts that give substance to the processes of figuring out what to do—facts such as that our children matter to us, and that we care about their well-being; that we care about our clan. Relative to these values, some solutions to social problems are better than others, *as a matter of fact*; relative to these values, practical policy decisions can be negotiated.

The hypothesis on offer is that what we humans call *ethics* or *morality* is a four-dimensional scheme for social behavior that is shaped by interlocking brain processes: (1) *caring* (rooted in attachment to kin and kith and care for their well-being),[11] (2) *recognition of others' psychological states* (rooted in the benefits of predicting the behavior others), (3) *problem-solving in a social context* (e.g., how we should distribute scarce goods, settle land disputes; how we should punish the miscreants), and (4) *learning social practices* (by positive and negative reinforcement, by imitation, by trial and error, by various kinds of conditioning, and by analogy). The simplicity of this framework does not mean its forms, variations, and neural mechanisms are simple. On the contrary, social life is stunningly complex, as is the brain that supports our social lives.

The human capacity for learning and for social problem-solving, constrained by the basic social urges, is the basis for what we commonly think of as social values. To be sure, in different contexts and cultures, particular articulations of those values may have different shapes and shades, even when the underlying social urges are shared. Values are, according to this hypothesis, more fundamental than rules. Various norms governing social life, reinforced by the reward/ punishment system, may eventually be articulated and even modified after deliberation, or they may remain as implicit, background knowledge about what "feels right."[12]

Reflecting on the necessities shaping cultures in vastly different conditions and on what social life might have been like for humans living in small groups 250,000 years ago leads us to questions of what distinguishes moral values from other values.[13] I generally shy away from trying to cobble together a precise definition of "moral," preferring to acknowledge that there is a spectrum of social behaviors, some of which involve matters of great seriousness, and tend to be called moral, such as enslaving captured prisoners or neglecting children, while others involve matters of more minor moment, such as conventions for behavior at a wedding. The boundaries of the concept "moral," like the boundaries of "house" or "vegetable," are fuzzy even when we can agree on prototypical cases, and this hampers precision in definition.[14] Moral values need not involve rules, though they sometimes do; they need not be explicitly stated, but may be implicitly picked up by children learning to get along in their social world, just as they implicitly pick up how to keep a fire going or how to tend goats.

While acknowledging the central role of cultural beliefs and practices in morality, my aim in this book is to examine the foundations of mammalian sociability in general, and human sociability in particular. I began this project because I wanted to understand what it is about the brains of highly social mammals that enables their sociability and thus to understand what grounds morality. I also wanted to understand variability in social temperament—in the urges to belong, to strongly empathize, and to form strong attachments. Though the approach through the various biological sciences may tell us a lot about the social platform, it is not, by any manner or means, the sum and substance of human morality. Nevertheless, coupled with hypotheses concerning cultural evolution and how culture can change the ecology of a species,[15] the neurobiological perspective may contribute to rounding out the portrait of human moral values that is being pieced together in the behavioral and brain sciences.

My contribution to the science of moral behavior is modest, because many questions in neuroscience and behavioral genetics are still unanswered. It is also very incomplete, because it focuses on the brain, not the recently developed culture in which modern brains live. It is limited because we cannot study the brains or behavior of early humans, nor those of our hominin ancestors.[16] Increasingly, we will learn about the genome of extinct hominins by recovering bits of DNA from bones, and some information will be garnered thereby. While acknowledging all these limitations, I hope that if my hypothesis is roughly on the right track, it may complement brain and behavioral research.

The core of the biological approach to human morality favored in this book is not new, though my particular way of synthesizing the data and encompassing the relevant philosophical tradition may be. The approach reaches back to Aristotle (384–322 BCE) and the great Chinese philosopher Mencius (fourth century BCE), to those sensible eighteenth-century Scots, David Hume and Adam Smith; it depends enormously on Charles Darwin. Advances in the biological and social sciences have made it possible to explore in earnest the connections between morality and the evolution of the mammalian brain that produced "the family way of life,"[17] and therewith, the wellspring of care and compassion that shapes the moral geography.

Briefly, the strategy for developing the central argument in the book is this: The next chapter will give a bit of background concerning the evolutionary constraints on social and moral behavior. The third chapter goes into detail on the evolution of the mammalian brain and how it supports caring, examining the role of hormones such as oxytocin. The fourth chapter looks more closely at cooperation, especially human cooperation, and data regarding the role of oxytocin in cooperation and trust. The fifth chapter on genes is cautionary, focusing on what is known, and not known, about "genes for" moral modules in the brain. The sixth chapter addresses the social importance of the capacity for attributing mental states, and the possible brain basis for such a capacity. In the seventh chapter, the matter of rules and the role of rules in moral behavior puts the discussion into a more traditional philosophical form. Religion and its relation to morality are the topics of the concluding chapter.

2. Brain-Based Values

Moral values ground a life that is a *social* life. At the root of human moral practices are the social desires; most fundamentally, these involve attachment to family members, care for friends, the need to belong. Motivated by these values, individually and collectively we try to solve problems that can cause misery and instability and threaten survival. Since our brains are organized to value self-welfare as well as welfare of kith and kin, conflicts frequently arise between the needs of self and the needs of others. Social problem-solving, grounded by social urges, leads to ways of handling these conflicts. Some solutions are more effective than others, and some may be socially unstable in the long run or as conditions change. Thus arise cultural practices, conventions, and institutions. As a child grows up within the social ecology of such practices, robust intuitions about right and wrong take root and flower.

Where do values come from? How did brains come to care about others? If my genes organize my brain to attend to my survival, to reproduce and pass on those genes, how can they organize my brain to value others? *Some*, but only some, of the neurobiology of this is beginning to be understood. First, however, the more fundamental question: how is it that brains care about *anything*?[1] To put it more tendentiously, how can neurons care? What does it mean for a system of neurons to care about or to value something? On these questions, we do know quite a lot, and the answers will launch us into the more complex domain of social caring.

In all animals, neural circuitry grounds self-caring and well-being. These are values in the most elemental sense. Lacking the motivation for self-preservation, an animal will neither long survive, nor likely reproduce. So evident is this, that the existence of social values, and of behavior directed toward the care of others, may seem deeply puzzling. Why do we, and other social mammals, care for others? This much we know: on average, such behavior must, either directly or indirectly, serve the fitness of the animals involved. Failing that, the behavior would be selected against, since it involves costs, including, most particularly, energy costs and sometimes risk to life and limb. That is, barring offsetting benefits for animals who incur the costs of "other-caring" behavior, over time the numbers of "other-caring" animals would dwindle, and the "self-caring" ones would increase in number. The population profile would change. What ultimately tells the accounting tale of costs and benefits is reproductive success; that is, the spread of genes through the population over many generations.

Neural mechanisms yielding cooperative behavior probably evolved many times. The nervous systems of insects and mammals are different in size and organization, and the mechanisms producing behavior that consists in caring for others will vary greatly between ants and humans, for example. Ants may show far greater levels of altruism than humans, in the sense of incurring cost to oneself in order to benefit the other. The sociability and voluntary association among individuals seen in humans, and the style of cooperation and other-caring, is mainly owed to evolutionary changes specific to the mammalian brain and the evolutionary pressures existing at the dawn of mammals, about

350 million years ago.[2] Within the mammalian family—about 5700 known species—all species are at least minimally social in that individuals come together to reproduce and mothers care for offspring. Some species, such as baboons and meerkats, are more highly social than others, such as black bears and orangutans, though typically solitary animals can be more social when abundance of resources reduces competition. For example, there are videos showing a polar bear, in the wild, companionably playing with a husky dog. Although strikingly different styles of social life have appeared, similarities in neural mechanisms owed to common organizational features in the mammalian brain help explain the existence of mammalian sociality in general.

A compelling line of evidence from neuroendocrinology, which studies hormone-brain interactions, suggests that in mammals (and quite possibly social birds), the neuronal organization whereby individuals see to their own well-being was modified to motivate new values—the well-being of certain others.[3] In early stages of the evolution of mammals, those *others* included only helpless offspring. Depending on ecological conditions and fitness considerations, strong caring for the well-being of offspring has in some mammalian species extended further to encompass kin or mates or friends or even strangers, as the circle widens. This widening of other-caring in social behavior marks the emergence of what eventually flowers into morality. The particular form a species' social life takes will depend greatly on how the species makes its living. For some species, group living is on average highly advantageous, especially in matters such as hunting and defense against predation; for others, such as bears, solitary foraging and self-defense suffice.

Oxytocin, a very ancient peptide (chain of amino acids), is at the hub of the intricate network of mammalian adaptations for caring for others, anchoring the many different versions of sociality that are seen, depending on the evolution of the lineage (see figure 2.1). Oxytocin is found in all vertebrates, but the evolution of the mammalian brain adapted oxytocin to new jobs in caring for offspring and eventually for wider forms of sociability.

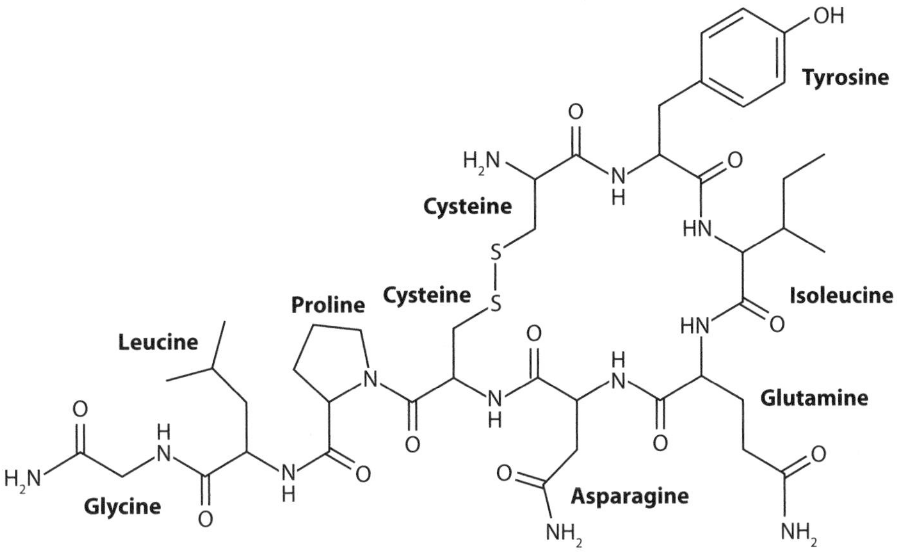

Figure 2.1. The molecular structure of oxytocin. Shown are its nine amino acids (cysteine occurs twice) linked by other molecules. By contrast, hemoglobin, the molecule in the blood that contains iron and carries oxygen, has about 500 amino acids. Hence oxytocin is considered a simple peptide (string of amino acids). Not shown is the three-dimensional structure of oxytocin.

Besides the new roles for oxytocin and other hormones, two additional interdependent evolutionary changes in the brain were crucial for the mammalian sociality that prefigured morality. The first involved modifications that gave rise to negative feelings of fear and anxiety in face of separation from or threat to the offspring, along with the motivation to take corrective action. In addition, pleasure and relief come when the parent is rejoined with the offspring or the threat has passed.[4] The second main modification was an increased capacity for learning, linked to pain and pleasure, that served an individual in acquiring detailed knowledge of the "ways" of others in the group. Expanded memory capacities greatly enhanced the animal's ability to anticipate trouble and to plan more effectively. These modifications support the urge to be together, as well as the development of a "conscience" tuned to local social practices; that is, a set of social responses, shaped by learning, that are strongly regulated by approval and disapproval, and by the emotions, more generally. More simply, mammals are motivated to learn social practices because the negative reward system, regulating pain, fear, and anxiety, responds to exclusion and disapproval, and the positive reward system responds to approval and affection.

In brief, the idea is that attachment, underwritten by the painfulness of separation and the pleasure of company, and managed by intricate neural circuitry and neurochemicals, is the neural platform for morality. In using the word *attachment*, I am adopting the terminology of neuroendocrinology, where *attachment* refers to the dispositions to extend care to others, to want to be with them, and to be distressed by separation.[5]

Archaeological evidence indicates that anatomically modern *Homo sapiens* existed in Africa about 300,000 years ago.[6] Evidence of culture, in the form of bone tools such as awls, barbed points, and polished points, as well as engraving using ochre, is dated about 75,000 years ago (found, for example, in the Blombos Cave, South Africa[7]). Remarkably, there is also some evidence of inter-group trade at this early date.[8] Curtis Marean of Arizona State University found even earlier evidence (about 110,00 years ago) in the South African region of Pinnacle Point of the use of high temperatures to "fire" the common substance silcrete to make especially sharp tools. This is an impressive cognitive achievement that involves a series of carefully executed steps: making a sand pit to bring the rock up to 350 degrees Celsius, holding the temperature steady for some time, and then slowly lowering the temperature.[9] Tools made of wood may have been common, but if so, in general they would not have been preserved for us to find.

Determining whether a fossil is consistent with modern human anatomy is difficult but possible, but determining whether the owner engaged in behavior considered modern is all but impossible. On this question, such scant evidence that does exist comes from archaeological discoveries of tools, objects, and body decorations, worked-dwelling remains, ritualized burial of the dead, and so forth. In the European sites to which a small group of Homo sapiens migrated, the technological finds, including cave art and tools, are dated about 40,000–50,000 years ago. Prior to the discoveries made at Blombos Cave and Pinnacle Point, these European archaeological finds were thought to mark the first appearance of human culture, suggesting to some anthropologists that genetic changes in early humans giving rise to a different brain must have occurred in the *Homo sapiens* that emigrated to Europe around 50,000 years ago. Both the presumed facts and the theory meant to explain them now appear unlikely, particularly given the Blombos Cave and Pinnacle Point discoveries dated around 75,000–110,000 years ago. These more ancient finds also make more tenuous the hunch that genes "for" language, more advanced technology, or morality emerged only around 50,000 years ago.

Relative to the finds so far, the basic point seems to be that culture was probably not a vastly greater factor in human social practices than in bonobo or baboon social practices, for example, until humans had been around for roughly 150,000 years. It seems likely that much of the social life of early humans, like human technological reliance on simple bone and stone tools, was probably rudimentary, involving small groups roving around Africa, Asia, and Europe. By *simple*, I mean simple relative to social life lived now, or even in ancient cities such as Athens, but certainly not simple relative to the social life of beavers or naked mole rats.

According to the archaeological record, the cranial capacity of humans living 250,000 years ago was roughly the same as ours (about 1300–1500 cubic centimeters), granting individual variation then, as now. (For comparison, chimpanzee brains are about 400 cc, and the Homo erectus brain was only about 800–1100 cc, based on cranial size.) Whether the details of neural anatomy were the same is of course unknown, since the brain rapidly decays after death. If we make the reasonable assumption that Middle Stone Age humans (300,000–50,000 years ago) had brains that, at birth, were pretty much like ours, at least in terms of social dispositions and problem-solving capacities, then any story of the neural underpinnings of human morality should apply to them as well. Cultural differences in moral practices—then and now—will abound, certainly, just as there are differences in technology and dwellings—then and now. Unlike our Middle Stone Age ancestors, contemporary humans regularly learn to read, ride bicycles, and play the guitar. Because learning involves structural changes in the brain, then of course the brains of those who have acquired these skills will be different from the brains of those who have not. In that sense my brain will be different from that of my ancient cousins circa 100,000 years ago. Nevertheless, relative to what we currently know, it is quite possible that they and I started out life with much the same neural equipment for sociality and cognition.

The assumption of rough similarity in cognitive and social capacities between us and our Stone Age relatives, lacking compelling evidence to the contrary, helps guard against injecting ideas from the modern era into *human nature*. It implies that we cannot assume that our Middle Stone Age ancestors in Africa and Europe had anything like the moral convictions of our contemporaries, despite sharing the fundamental platform.[10] Thus when the philosopher Susan Neiman points to what she sees as the deep human need for moral purpose, of the yearning of humanity for moral progress, her insightful remarks probably apply only to humans living in the fairly recent past, and then, perhaps, only to those who had the prosperity, longevity, leisure, and cultural background to reflect on moral purpose.[11] Such yearnings for moral progress might be culturally fostered, as are the ideas of technological or scientific progress.

It would not be surprising to me if, for much of human history, our ancestors were too busy with birth and death, food and shelter, to give a great deal of thought to moral progress, though of course we do not know what they did in their spare time. Just as the brain did not evolve to read, but to do complex pattern recognition to help guide action, so it is entirely possible it did not evolve to favor universal human rights, or trial by jury. This point does not mean that the idea of moral progress does not motivate us now, but it does suggest we need to be cautious about ascribing such values as a yearning for moral progress to early *Homo sapiens*, and hence to our basic nature here and now.

Compared to other mammals, humans have a very large brain relative to body size. In some imprecise sense, we are smarter than other mammals: we have greater cognitive flexibility, and a greater capacity for abstraction and for long-term planning, and we show an especially strong ability and inclination to imitate.[12] What exactly is conferred by larger brain size and how it contributes to intelligence, however, is anything but clear.[13] Disappointingly, the link between expanded cortex and intelligence is not well understood, though it is known that the prefrontal cortex is important in decision-making, impulse control, and attributing goals and perceptions to others.[14] Speculations linking intelligence to brain size are plentiful, but until more is known about brain function and organization, these are rightly regarded as nice stories.

Humans have developed highly intricate languages and rich cultures, and hence our sociality and our systems of ethical values have become correspondingly complex. It appears probable that our technology and art—and one might guess, language—were relatively primitive for at least 200,000 years. Stone hand axes, for example, seem to have been the only tool ever made and used by Neanderthals, and the only tool of *Homo sapiens* for about 200,000 years or so. Spear technology seems so obvious to us, yet for 200,000 years, it may not have occurred to anybody. Putting spoken words into writing, for yet another example, seems utterly obvious to us, yet writing and reading were not invented by *Homo sapiens* until perhaps 5400 years ago. Consequently, we cannot assume that having a big brain made inventing and innovating, either in technological or social domains, an obvious or inevitable business.

Science journalist Matt Ridley argues that once bartering and swapping began, once various artifacts, such as harpoons or body ornaments, were traded among groups, artifactual and social innovation accelerated.[15] Evidence for exchange of goods between groups dates to about 100,000 years ago, which implies that humans did not engage in exchange for some 200,000 years. The unique value in swapping what I have for the different things that you have was, in Ridley's view, a turning point in human economies that marked the beginning of the long, slow development of technologies and labor specialization. If I make lots of spears but have no nets, and then trade some of my spears for some of your nets, suddenly my toolbox has doubled. Consequently, my opportunities for getting food have greatly increased.

As Ridley's hypothesis explains, swap and barter rewarded innovation and specialization, which in turn motivated yet more swap and barter, inspiring yet more innovation and specialization. Likely the earliest steps in barter were hardly recognizable as such, but somehow the advantages of swapping or exchanging were recognized by some people, for the practice spread and became ever more sophisticated. This positive feedback loop helped foster the creation of social practices in trade that increased the chances of prosperity for the innovators and swappers.

Just as writing was invented without a "writing gene," so barter and trade were probably stumbled upon and improved upon, without support of a "barter gene." The capacity for problem-solving, whatever that really involves in terms of brain circuitry, allows for the emergence of novel behaviors, without the aid of new genes.

Cultural history and evolution have been the focus of elegant empirical and theoretical work in the social sciences.[16] An important theme emerging from this work concerns the dynamics of cultural evolution; for example, that cultural evolution can happen much faster than biological evolution, and that cultural institutions can constitute a change in ecological conditions that in turn can alter selection pressures.[17] The advantages of barter and exchange of unlike goods (my spears for your nets) is an example of a change in social ecology that alters selection pressures by expanding the domain of resources available. Snaring gophers with twine, for example, is a lot faster and more reliable than trying to sneak up and club them.

The slow shift from a hunter-gatherer to an agrarian mode of subsistence that began about 10,000 years ago was a cultural transformation that wrought many changes in the conditions of social life. Reliable supplies of milk and meat from goats, as well as the harvest of grains and vegetables, diminished somewhat the uncertainties of depending solely on foraging. One of the more important social changes was the aggregation into larger groups that included many non-kin. Life in a larger group gave rise to new opportunities for improving well-being, as well as new forms of within-group and between-group competition, along with new kinds of social problems to be solved.

Evidence for some genetic changes within the last 10,000 years does exist, but so far these changes pertain not to brain circuitry, cognition, or social temperament, but to properties that are arguably more amenable to evolutionary change without triggering a deleterious cascade of changes. An important example is the genetic change that allowed adult humans to digest animal milks. Mammalian babies would not be able to live on milk if it weren't for lactase, an enzyme needed to digest milk. In Stone Age humans lactase petered out at weaning (as it does in most mammals) and with it, the ability to digest milk. But about 10,000 years ago—around the time that goats and cows were domesticated—humans who happened to carry a gene that continued to produced lactase into adulthood (lactase persistence) had a selective advantage because they could digest milk. Thus in herding populations the numbers of adult humans with lactase persistence gradually increased.[18] At least four different genetic changes are known to be related to lactase persistence, and they appeared at different times in Europe and in Africa, probably correlated with the local adoption of herding and milking.[19]

Claims for genetic changes related to social and cognitive behavior are much more difficult to demonstrate, and though intriguing, remain conjectural. The stories are possibly true, but science needs evidence for belief. Keep in mind that genes make proteins, and that there are very long causal routes between proteins and brain circuitry, and further long causal routes between brain circuitry and the environment, which in turn affects gene expression and proteins. Genes are part of genetic networks, and these networks interact with the environment in complex ways. There is no doubt that our genes are massively important in what we are and for the variability among us, but from that observation, nothing very specific can be concluded, such as that there is a "gene for" fairness or religion or wanderlust. To be sure, it would be quite wrong to suppose that changes in the human genome that affect brain structure ground to a halt about 200,000 years ago. Nevertheless, demonstrating a causal relation between genes and behavior, and then showing that the gene and the behavior were selected for, cannot be achieved merely by telling a fetching story. What is stunning about humans is how easily we learn such a vast range of things, things that, given the culture, we would not have had an opportunity to learn 200,000 years ago. Within a technologically and institutionally rich culture, the things we learn often make us smart, relative to those in a simpler culture. If making spears by tying hand axes to sturdy branches seems obvious to me, or if writing down what you owe me from our exchange seems obvious to me, that is because my culture makes me smart in those ways. Would I, had I lived in Africa 200,000 years ago, have concocted the idea of a spear for throwing instead of a hand axe for tearing? I am inclined to doubt it.

As a brief illustration, I will mention that about twenty years ago I took ten adventurous undergraduates from the University of California–San Diego on a rafting trip in the Arctic, from the headwaters of the Firth River to the Beaufort Sea and on to Herschel Island in the Arctic Ocean. These were students at the top of their classes, preparing for medical school, graduate school, and business school, but they were all entirely naïve about trekking in the wild. On the second day out, our Inuit guide quietly took me aside after dinner and asked me whether these were especially stupid students. The point was, they did the dumbest things when trying to put up tents, prepare food, load the rafts, get in and out of the raft, and so on. The things that were second nature to our guide and his young children, such as always checking the sky to see about weather changes, were skills of which the students were completely ignorant. They did quickly learn, however, which he appreciated, and after seven days he generously taught them how to stalk a herd of musk ox.

But Surely Only Humans Are Moral?

As we consider the differences and similarities between the brains of humans and other mammals, a background question comes to the fore: do only humans have moral values, or can other animals also be said to have moral values, albeit ones suited to their own social organization and ecology? Because there are common underlying motifs and mechanisms in the behavior of social mammals in general, the question of whether nonhumans have moral values is anything but straightforward. "Human-style" morality, moreover, is not a single set of moral values, given the variability in what human cultures adduce as their moral values. Some cultures accept infanticide for the disabled or unwanted, others consider it morally abhorrent; some consider a mouthful of the killed enemy's flesh a requirement for a courageous warrior, others consider it barbaric.

Although attachment may be the platform for morality, there is no simple set of steps—no deductive operation, no exactly applicable rule—to take us from "I care, I value" to the best solution to specific moral problems, especially those problems that arise within complex cultures. Pretty obviously, social problem-solving is a messy practical business within an individual brain, where many interacting factors push, pull, compete, and constrain the decision the brain settles on. Some constraints take priority over others; some factors will be conscious, others not; some can be articulated, some not. In general, decision-making is a constraint-satisfaction business, and when it goes well, we say that rationality has prevailed.[20] Even more complex than individual decision-making is the business of addressing social problems within a social group, where competing interests, beliefs, temperaments, and traditions constrain the decision the group settles on, each individual brain in the mix having its own set of internal constraints.[21] Moral progress, where it is embodied in institutions and laws, seems to depend greatly on negotiation, institutional history, and small-p politics.

Reflecting on the differences between the social behavior of humans on the one hand, and on the other, that of chimpanzees, baboons, orcas, elephants, meerkats, and marmosets, it may be most useful to shelve the assumption that there are exactly two kinds of morality: human and animal. The problem with the assumption is that each social species appears to be unique in various respects, even while having features in common. Bonobos, uniquely it seems, use sex as a means of reducing social tension; chimpanzees and baboons do not; gibbons will socialize with a neighboring group, gorillas and lemurs will not. Humans use laughter as a means of reducing tension, and in chimpanzees play-panting and the accompanying "play face" seems also to serve such a role,[22] but baboons and lemurs do not appear to have a homologue of this behavior. In chimpanzees, females reaching reproductive age leave the troop to find a new home, but in baboons, it is the males that leave at maturity. The chimp pattern seems to be the pattern also in some hunter-gatherer societies such as the Inuit of the Arctic. Such behavioral patterns affect many aspects of ranking and hierarchy. In meerkats, the alpha female will kill babies of a less dominant female, and drive her out of the group; by contrast, in baboons, all fertile females in the troop produce babies. Moreover, within a species there can be local styles (perhaps *norms*, even though not formulated in language).[23]

In small groups of hunter-gathering humans, such as the Inuit before the twentieth century, it was not uncommon to capture women from the camps of other tribes, undoubtedly a practice that served, albeit without conscious intent, to diversify the gene pool. Those in modern western societies who favor a rules approach to morality would likely condemn the practice as showing a violation of moral rules. I would not find this an easy judgment, however, since the alternative—in-breeding—has hazards I would not want to have visited upon the Inuit, and would not have wanted for myself, were I an Inuit living in the Arctic in the pre-European period. Within our own culture, there is often disagreement about the evaluation of an act. In 1972 bush pilot Martin Hartwell, courageously agreeing to fly a mercy flight despite a bad weather, tragically crashed the bush plane. His passengers included an Inuit child who desperately needed an appendectomy and a nurse along to care for him. The nurse died on impact, and eventually the child died as well. With two broken legs, starving and near death after many weeks of waiting in vain for rescue, Hartwell consumed the leg of his friend, the dead nurse. Eventually, after 31 days in the bitter cold, Hartwell was rescued. On cannibalism in such extreme circumstances, opinion varies greatly, and I am doubtful that there is a uniquely correct answer, even when all the details of the story are known. Many well-fed people are horrified at the prospect of eating their dog, but the traditional Inuit are comparably horrified at the idiocy of starving to death when eating a dog would keep life going until game was found. As we all know well, rational people may disagree about the best way to handle taxation, or education of the young, or when to wage preemptive wars. Often there are better or worse choices, but no uniquely right choice; in such cases, constraint satisfaction does its business—balancing and harmonizing and settling on a suitable decision.

The foregoing also suggests it may be wise to avoid a related assumption according to which only humans have "true" morality; other animals, according to this view, may be complex and social, but strictly speaking they are *amoral*. In part, what you say here depends on whose *strict speaking* rules the ways we use words. But there is no "meaning czar" whose opinion rules the use of words. If you define words such that true morality requires language and linguistically formulated rules, well then, yes, you can infer that only humans have true morality. But what progress is achieved by such semantic stipulation? And anyhow, *why* define "true morality" as requiring language? Some, such as the contemporary moral philosopher Christine Korsgaard, adhere to a rather different argument: only humans are genuinely rational, morality depends on rationality, and hence nonhuman animals are not moral.[24] Because many species of birds and mammals display good examples of problem-solving and planning, this claim about rationality looks narrow and under-informed.[25]

That nonhuman mammals have social values is obvious; they care for juveniles, and sometimes mates, kin, and affiliates; they cooperate, they may punish, and they reconcile after conflict.[26] We could engage in a semantic wrangle about whether these values are really *moral* values, but a wrangle about words is apt to be unrewarding. Of course only humans have *human* morality. But that is not news, simply a tedious tautology. One might as well note that only marmosets have *marmoset* morality, and so on down the line. We can agree that ants are not moral in the way humans are, and that baboon and bonobo social behavior is much closer to our own. With no home movies to give us clues, we do not know whether the social behavior of other hominins—for example, *Homo erectus* or *Homo neanderthalensis* or *Homo heidelbergensis*—was very close to the social behavior of modern humans. Perhaps we can leave it at that, pending deeper scientific understanding.

3. Caring and Caring For

What is going on in the brain such that an animal cares about others, or expresses *social* values? According to the hypothesis on offer, it is the neurochemistry of attachment and bonding in mammals that yields the central explanatory element.[1] Therefore, to understand the brain-based platform for social values, we first have to consider the more fundamental question, which will lead us back to social values: how is it that brains care about *anything*? To put it somewhat differently, how can *neurons* value something?

The first and most fundamental part of the story concerns self-preservation.[2] All nervous systems are organized to take care of the basic survival of the body they are part of. From an evolutionary perspective, the general point is straightforward: self-caring is selected over self-neglect. Animals that fail at self-preserving behavior have no chance to pass on their genes, whereas animals that succeed in keeping their bodies healthy have a shot at passing on their genes. For an animal to survive, the world must be traversed to find energy, water, and whatever else is needed to keep the body going. Pain and fear are survival signals, indicating the need for corrective behavior. Different kinds of pain signal different avenues of behavioral correction.

These general observations raise questions concerning neural mechanisms: how does a mouse, for example, know that it should find food, or scurry into a burrow, or make a nest? How are behavioral decisions serving well-being achieved by neurons?

The rough answer is that the neurons in the brainstem and hypothalamus of the mouse monitor the mouse's *internal milieu*—the inner state of its body relative to the parameters that matter for survival. When a particular need is detected, a motivational emotion is generated. In the mouse—and in us—brainstem and hypothalamic neurons regulate body temperature, glucose levels, blood pressure, heart rate, and carbon dioxide levels. *Homeostasis* is the process whereby the internal environment of the organism is regulated to stay close to the range needed for survival. And pain, as neuroscientist Bud Craig has observed, is a homeostatic emotion.[3] We are all familiar with changes in the internal milieu that signal the need to redress an imbalance: the panic when oxygen is cut off, the unpleasantness of being cold, the sensation of thirst, of nausea, and the pain of extreme hunger. These are accompanied by distinct urges—to seek warmth, water, food; to vomit, run away, snuggle, and so forth.

Using perceptual cues such as odors and sounds, the mouse's subcortical brain also assesses risk and opportunity in the outside world. In mice, the smell of seeds provokes approach behavior; in a male mouse, the smell associated with a female in estrus provokes courting behavior. A male mouse entering a new territory where he smells the urine of another male mouse will be inclined to go elsewhere.

In us, the fear induced by a snarling dog or the panic induced by unpredicted smoke are unmistakable and unpleasant feelings. These life-relevant feelings are integrated, and appropriate movement is coordinated, by subcortical structures in the brainstem and the hypothalamus, as well as in the insular cortex and the cingulate cortex (figure 3.1). Mechanisms in the sympathetic nervous system adjust the body

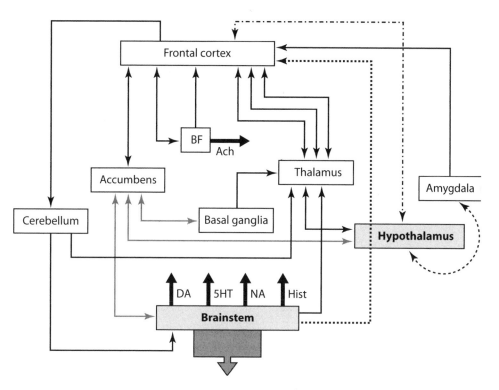

Figure 3.1. This schematically illustrates some of the subcortical structures and their connection to the cortex. Notice in particular the rich pathways between the frontal areas and the subcortical areas, including those involving reward (accumbens) and fear (amygdala). The hypothalamus is broadly connected to many structures, typically in a bidirectional manner. From the brainstem emerge four neuronal projection systems with distinct neurochemicals, each system reaching very broadly into many areas. The four neurochemicals, sometimes called neuromodulators, are serotonin (5HT), noradrenaline (NA), dopamine (DA), and histamine (Hist). Based on Josef Parvizi, "Corticocentric Myopia: Old Bias in New Cognitive Sciences," *Trends in Cognitive Sciences* 13, no. 8 (2009):354–59. (To see the location of the amygdala in 3-space, go to http://commons.wikimedia.org/wiki/File:Amygdala_small.gif.)

for "fight or flight," and when the threat has passed, other mechanisms in the parasympathetic system restore the blood pressure and heart rate to the energetically less costly state of "rest and digest." Moreover, the circuitry is sensitive to priorities, so that fear of a looming predator trumps hunger for the tasty nut or lust for the ready female.

Integrating signals from both the inner milieu and the body surface, the brainstem-limbic circuitry is the foundational organization serving self-preservation, and therewith a minimal sense of self.[4] Maintaining the health and welfare of the body constitutes the neurobiological scaffolding for higher levels of self-representation, such as the sense of self as a person belonging to a social group and having special bonds to special individuals.[5]

In the most basic sense, therefore, *caring* is a ground-floor function of nervous systems. Brains are organized to seek well-being, and to seek relief from ill-being. Thus, in a perfectly straightforward way, the circuitry for self-maintenance and the avoidance of pain is the source of the most basic values—the values of being alive and of well-being. For frogs and salmon and newts, this sort of caring is pretty much all there is. Even so, this level of integration, highly conserved in all vertebrates, is exquisitely complicated.

Selection pressure for self-caring is clear-cut, even when the underlying circuitry is obscured by complexity. How can caring for *others* be explained? As proposed in chapter 2, the core idea is that in mammals, evolutionary adjustments in the emotional, endocrine, stress, and reward/punishment systems effectively *extend* the range of individuals whose well-being the animal cares about, at least for a certain set of survival-relevant behaviors. Thus the mother rat behaves as though the newborn pups are included in her basic homeostatic ambit—they must be fed, cleaned, and kept warm, as well as protected from the assorted dangers of the world, just as *she* must keep herself fed, warm, clean, and safe from the dangers of the world. When the pups are threatened, their well-being matters to her in somewhat the same way her own well-being matters to her, and corrective behavior is taken. Pain and fear, her homeostatic emotions that are both feeling and motivation, are triggered when the well-being of her pups is at risk. It is as though the golden circle of *me* expands to include *my* helpless pups (see figure 3.2).[6]

True enough, a wolf or a rat will normally abandon her pups when the threat is perceived to be overwhelming and she needs to save herself

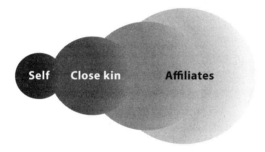

Figure 3.2. A cartoon depicting the spheres of caring. Circuitry serving one's own survival and well-being is modified in mammals to embrace one's babies. In social mammals, the embrace may include close kin, close friends, other group members, and even strangers, typically with decreasing intensity depending on the degree of attachment.

even if the pups cannot be saved. So the extension of her homeostatic ambit to include the pups still allows for recognition of the distinction between self and dearly beloved others. Human parents similarly confronting an overwhelming foe may elect to save themselves, though sometimes the motivation to save the juvenile can lead to the self-sacrifice of the parent. Human behavior in such dire circumstances will also depend on many other factors, including the nature of the calamity, individual temperament, sociocultural background, and the existence of other offspring. These are very powerful systems that interweave with but go well beyond the very powerful system for self-preservation. The "going beyond" is not haphazard, but is systematically related to the well-being of others, especially those who are kin.[7]

The crucial steps that lead from *only* self-caring, to the variety of kinds of sociality (*other-caring*) typical of mammals, depend on the neural-and-body mechanisms that "maternalize" the female mammalian brain, which in turn depend on the neuropeptides oxytocin (OXT) and arginine vasopressin (AVP), along with other hormones. Almost certainly these mechanisms were not initially selected to serve any broader social purposes, but merely to ensure that the female had the resources and motivation to suckle, defend, and, more generally, to devote herself to the welfare of her helpless juveniles until they were independent. Mammals whose circuitry outfitted them for offspring care had more of their offspring survive than those inclined to offspring neglect.

Once in place, however, the modification that yields caring for others that *are* offspring could be further modified, perhaps in quite minor ways, to yield caring for others that are *not* offspring, but whose well-being is consequential for the well-being of oneself and one's offspring. Depending on the species and its selection pressures, different social arrangements would be selected for, and many other brain mechanisms would be put in play. Thus in a wolf pack or a beaver colony, there is only one breeding pair; in baboon troops and orca pods, all the fertile females breed. Ringtail lemurs are matrilineal; the females are dominant with respect to the males, and mate with multiple males. In river otters and grizzly bears, the group consists of a female and her pups, and the female breeds with any suitable male that courts her appropriately. In rhesus monkeys, the babies are attached only to the mother, while in titi monkeys, they are more strongly attached to the father than to the mother. This is just a tiny sample of the range of social patterns found among mammals, but underlying them all are probably different arrangements of receptors for oxytocin and other hormones and neurochemicals.

Neuroscientists Porges and Carter raise the question why OXT and AVP should be suited to their special roles in the mammalian brain.[8] In answering, they point out that these peptides are extremely ancient (at least 700 million years, predating mammals), and are involved in the regulation of water and minerals in the bodies of terrestrial animals generally. An evolutionarily earlier version of oxytocin and vasopressin—vasotocin—plays a role in amphibian mating behavior and is important in egg-laying. Long before the appearance of mammals, vasotocin was in the reproductive game. In mammals, the regulation of water and minerals became ever more sophisticated, since during pregnancy, the female needed to grow a placenta, and an amniotic sac filled with fluid in which the babies develop, and after birth she needed to produce milk for the babies.[9] This gives us a broad hint about why OXT and AVP lent themselves to evolutionary tinkering in mammalian reproduction, and why homologues of these peptides are important in avian sociality. As biologist James Hunt has observed, "Sociality, like multicellularity, has appeared numerous times, in diverse taxa, and reached many different levels of integration."[10] Not all forms can be assumed to involve OXT and AVP, and for those that do, the ways in which they do may differ.

How, at the neural level, is *attachment* achieved in mammals? In order to move forward on that question, we first need to explore the attachment story in more detail.

Family Values:
Belonging and Wanting to Belong

In all pregnant mammals, humans included, the placenta of the fetus releases a variety of hormones into the mother's bloodstream that have the effect of "maternalizing" her brain.[11] These hormones, including progestin, estrogen, and prolactin, act mainly on neurons in subcortical structures.[12] In rodents and cats, for example, this causes the pregnant female to eat more, to prepare a nest for the expected litter, and to find a place reckoned as safe to give birth. Human females too respond to a "nesting" urge as the time for delivery draws near, and (as I can personally attest) begin energetically to house-clean and finalize preparations for the new baby. OXT production is upregulated (made more plentiful) during pregnancy; at birth, release of OXT plays a role in causing the uterus to contract. OXT is also essential in the ejection of milk during lactation. In the brain, the release of OXT triggers full maternal behavior, including preoccupation with the infants, suckling, and keeping the infants warm, clean, and safe. In humans, maternal behavior may also be triggered by a baby a woman adopts as her own, and the attachment can be every bit as powerful as attachment to a baby carried and delivered.[13] This likely also involves release of oxytocin. Aunties of meerkat infants also respond in this way. Other mammals, with babies of their own, have been known to nurture the babies of another species, as when a dog contentedly suckles a pig or a kitten.

The *endogenous opiates*, those opium-like molecules cooked up by our own brain, probably also play a crucial role in maternal bonding, and the suckling female gets the reward of pleasure from opiates released during lactation. In my experience, I would say that lactation is pleasurable and calming, but it does not make you "high" in any recognizable sense. Rhesus monkey mothers who are given naloxone, a chemical that blocks the receptors for the opioids and so blocks their effect, show indifference to their babies, and tend to neglect them. Ewes injected with naloxone will actively reject their lambs. Although there are complicating social factors, human female heroin addicts tend to neglect or abandon their infants in unusually high numbers. In addicts, presumably, the modest effect of the endogenous opiates is swamped by the overwhelming effects of relatively large amounts of heroin,[14] though abnormalities in OXT levels may play a role as well. Cocaine-abusing human mothers, for example, have lower levels of OXT than non-addict controls, and display less maternal behavior.[15] Normally, however, tending to the infant is rewarding; it feels good. By contrast, anxiety levels rise when the infant is crying, taken away, or suffering, and this feels very bad.

That brings us to pain, or more broadly, negative affect, which is a central player in the emergence of mammalian social behavior.[16] Pain, though it may seem simple enough as experienced, is supported by astonishingly complicated anatomy, with many different specializations, components, neurochemicals, pathways, and connections.[17] In addition to the changes involving oxytocin, the mammalian system for negative affect—pain, fear, panic, anxiety—was also modified. In all vertebrates, fear, anxiety, and physical pain are registered as "protect-myself" warning signals in the brainstem and hypothalamus. These changes lead to a repertoire of corrective behavior by self-preservation circuitry. Evolutionary modifications to these basic systems ensure that mammals respond to threat and injury to offspring as well as to themselves. The feelings and responses engaged for the *protect-myself* tactics are also engaged for *protect-mine* tactics.

A signature feature of the mammalian brain is the cortex: a regularly organized six-layer sheet that constitutes the outer rind of the cerebral hemispheres (see figure 3.3).[18] This amazing evolutionary invention packs a lot of processing structure into a confined space, cleverly using a *small-world* organization to maximize processing power without loss of accessibility; that is, there are dense connections locally, sparse connections to distant regions, but by virtue of well-connected neighbors, any area can reach other areas in a few steps. In our story, the modification of particular interest concerns the cortical elaboration of the representation of pain, and in particular, the pain that occurs during separation from or threat to loved ones.

Pain, as neuroscientist A. D. (Bud) Craig ruefully acknowledges, is an enigma. Still, major discoveries in the last fifteen years, many by Craig and his colleagues, have corrected some old and honored misconceptions, and made pain in all its oddities a little less mysterious.[19] By classing pain as a homeostatic emotion, rather than as a sensation such as pressure, Craig means to emphasize its central role in the wider set of mechanisms for self-preservation. This makes for a contrast with the role of vision or audition, which are mainly devoted to representing the external world but do not automatically carry motivational "feel" in the way that a burn, for example, does. The contrast is a matter of degree, of course, since ultimately vision and audition also serve self-preservation—sometimes just a little less directly. As with thirst or cold, pain signals coming from the body's innards or muscles or joints or its surface activate the felt need for correction. As part of the dynamical processes for maintaining homeostasis, the sensory aspect of pain can vary even when the stimulus is unchanged; for

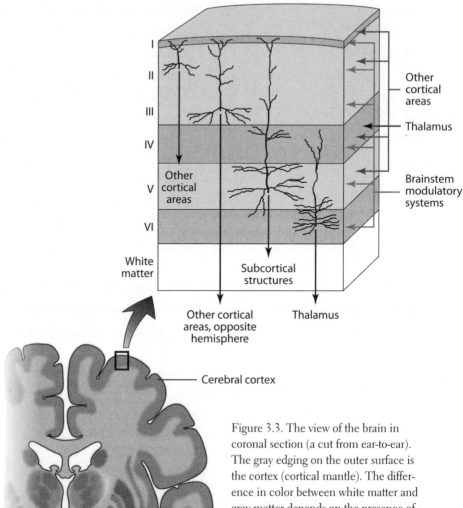

Figure 3.3. The view of the brain in coronal section (a cut from ear-to-ear). The gray edging on the outer surface is the cortex (cortical mantle). The difference in color between white matter and gray matter depends on the presence of myelin, which consists of fat-rich cells that wrap themselves around the axons of neurons, providing a kind of insulation resulting in faster signal transmission. Gray matter lacks myelin. The cutaway depicts the cortex's laminar organization and highly regular architecture. Not conveyed is the density of neurons: there are about 100,000 neurons in one cubic millimeter of cortical tissue, with about one billion synaptic connections between neurons. Adapted from A. D. Craig, "Pain Mechanisms: Labeled Lines versus Convergence in Central Processing," *Annual Review of Neuroscience* 26 (2003):1–30, and E. G. Jones, "Laminar Distribution of Cortical Efferent Cells," in *Cellular Components of the Cerebral Cortex*, ed. A. Peters and E. G. Jones (New York: Plenum, 1984), vol. 1, pp. 521–53.

example, soldiers shot in the heat of battle may feel no pain until safely in the field hospital, just as they may feel no thirst or hunger either.

As shown in figure 3.4, the central pain system in humans arises in a region of the spinal cord called lamina I, where signals concerning injury (nociception) are received from body tissues and organs. The pathway carries these signals up the spinal cord, into the brainstem, where there is cross-talk with regions regulating homeostatic responses, and then proceeds to specific regions of the thalamus. This system, known as the *spinothalamic tract*, allows for very precise localization of nociceptive signals, and for distinct kinds of painful feelings—a sharp hurt versus a burning sensation versus the sorrow of loss. Cortically, two places play a crucial role in pain processing: the *insula* (tucked in under the frontal lobe and easy to miss) appears essential for the nastiness of painful experiences—the qualitatively negative aspects —while the *anterior cingulate cortex* (ACC), to which it is connected, dominates the motivational (*do* something) aspect of pain. The insula, shown in figure 3.5, serially integrates body signals to yield a full state-of-my-body report.

Signals first reach the posterior part of the insula, and then appear to be reprocessed through a series of stages from the back to the front of the insula, probably ascending in the complexity and integration of what is represented. The insula appears to represent state-of-me and state-of-mine, as it integrates signals from all over the body and brain. When something is registered as being amiss, such as encroaching cold or an impending attack, it responds with distress signals, motivating redress. Consistent with the neuroanatomy, patients with front-temporal dementia, involving destruction of neurons in the insula, exhibit a striking loss of empathic responses as well as a diminution of experienced pain.

The region at the top of the processing hierarchy—the anterior insula—seems to be unique to primates, and is more highly developed in humans than in other primates.[20] What these differences mean in terms of differences in capacity is not established, but they may bear upon the representational complexity of state-of-me and state-of-mine,

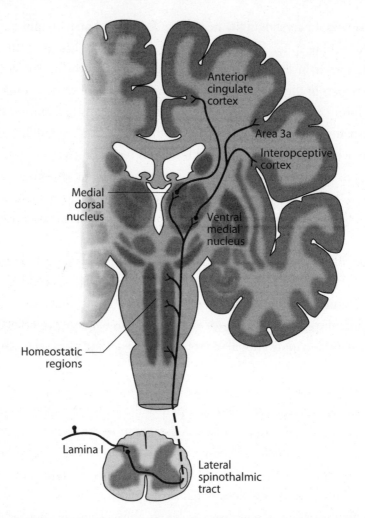

Figure 3.4. The drawing depicts the dominant pain pathway in the human brain and spinal cord as would be seen in a coronal section. The cortex and other gray matter structures (mainly the bodies of neurons) are shown as darker gray; white matter (mainly myelinated axons of neurons) are depicted as lighter gray. Notice that the lateral spinothalamic tract makes connections in the brainstem with the region regulating homeostasis, and then goes on to make synaptic connections in two distinct nuclei (gray matter regions) in the thalamus. One thalamic nucleus projects to the anterior insula (interoceptive cortex), containing a representation of the physiological state of the body, and to somatosensory cortex (area 3a); the other nucleus sends neurons to the ACC (anterior cingulate cortex). From A. D. Craig, "Pain Mechanisms: Labeled Lines versus Convergence in Central Processing," *Annual Review of Neuroscience* 26 (2003):1–30. Reprinted with permission.

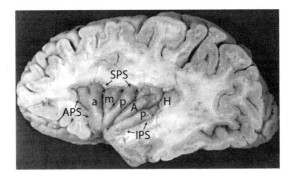

Figure 3.5. An anatomical photograph showing the insula in the left hemisphere. The insula has been exposed by dissecting away parts of the frontal lobe, temporal lobe, and parietal lobe. The insula can also be exposed without dissection by lifting the frontal lobe away from the temporal lobe. (A gyrus is a hill; a sulcus is a gully; the geography is the effect of folding as the growing brain is constrained within the boundaries of the skull. The landmarks are roughly, but only roughly, similar across individuals) a,m,p: anterior, middle, and posterior gyri of the anterior insula; A, P: anterior and posterior gyri of the posterior insula; APS: anterior periinsular sulcus; SPS: superior periinsular sulcus; IPS: inferior periinsular sulcus; H: Heschel gyrus. Reproduced with permission from Thomas P. Naidich et al., "The Insula: Anatomic Study and MR Imaging Display at 1.5 T," *American Journal of Neuroradiology* 25 (2004):226.

perhaps allowing for prolonged sorrow for a loss, or for more abstract representations of possible future states of me-and-mine.[21]

Because humans have social brains, our more generalized pain system makes us feel awful not just when our own well-being is threatened, but when the well-being of loved ones is threatened. Infant mammals are frightened when separated from those to whom they are attached, and make distress calls. This is a good thing, since they cannot feed and defend themselves, and need their mother or father.[22] As well, mammalian mothers, and in some species, fathers, feel anxious and awful when they hear their offspring make distress calls—also a good thing, and for the corresponding reason: their babies need them. Both the insula and the ACC respond to physical pain, but they also respond to social pain triggered by separation, exclusion, or disapproval, and to pain resulting from errors and poor predictions.[23]

When a mammalian mother is successful in making the infant safe and content, endogenous opiates as well as OXT are released, both in the brain of the contented infant, and in the brain of the relieved mother. Being together feels good. Humans know what this feels like even if we do not know anything about oxytocin or the endogenous opiates.

Feelings of remorse, guilt, and shame are typical in most, but not all, humans after having injured another. Psychopaths, though they know the social importance of expressing remorse in a courtroom, actually feel none, even after causing terror, mutilation, and death. Psychopaths are people who may be cunning and charming in the social world but who are without conscience, and tend not to form strong attachments.[24] Studies of psychopaths (the terms *psychopath* and *sociopath* are often used interchangeably) have allowed for the synthesis of quite precise criteria for the diagnosis.[25] Individuals diagnosed as psychopaths typically have six or more felonies in their criminal record, are unlikely to form long-term relationships, are manipulative and deceptive, and tend not to have deep feelings, positive or negative, about most things. Ted Bundy, who confessed to thirty murders between 1974 and 1978, and engaged in torture and necrophilia, was a classic psychopath; utterly without remorse or guilt at his actions, yet by all accounts attractive and charming. By contrast, Charles Manson, a cult leader convicted of conspiracy to commit the Tate and LaBianca murders in Los Angeles in 1969, was clearly delusional, imagining he was leading a revolution for the benefit of the people.

Are the brains of psychopaths different? It seems so. The data available so far suggest important differences between the brains of psychopaths and those of healthy controls in those areas regulating emotions, impulses, and social responses. Specifically, the *paralimbic* regions of the brain are different in psychopaths both anatomically (smaller in size) and functionally (lower levels of activity in emotional learning and decision-making tasks).[26] Paralimbic areas include those one would expect to be implicated: subcortical structures regulating

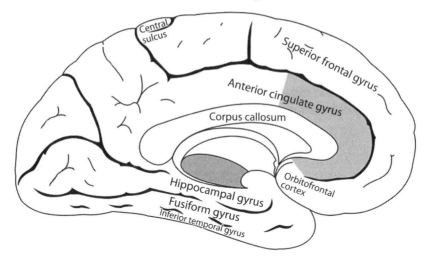

Figure 3.6. Sketch of the human brain showing the location of the anterior cingulate cortex, orbitofrontal cortex, (so-called because it is located just above the orbits of the eyes) hippocampal gyrus, superior frontal gyrus, inferior temporal gyrus, fusiform gyrus, and corpus callosum (the main connecting pathway between the two hemispheres). Based on Wikimedia Commons (http://commons.wikimedia.org/w/index .php?title=Special%3ASearch&search=anterior+cingulate).

emotional responses, such as the amygdala and the septum, structures related to memory (hippocampal areas); and the cortical areas known to be involved in social interactions, including feeling social pain and pleasure (the insula, ACC, orbital frontal cortex, and lateral temporal lobe; see figure 3.6).[27]

Twin and family studies suggest a heritability of psychopathy in the range of about 70%; childhood conditions such as abuse and neglect may contribute to those who are genetically disposed.[28] Because a significant proportion of the prison population—perhaps 30–40%—score high on the psychopathy criteria, and because psychopaths can be both deceptive and destructive, this is a social disorder of great concern. Psychopathy also reminds us of the importance of negative affect in social intercourse—its crucial role in learning appropriate social behavior, in suppressing antisocial actions, and in developing a conscience. If you feel no social pain, then a life-destroying mutilation has about the same significance as a lighthearted prank.[29]

Because human brains have large prefrontal and limbic regions, we need not respond rigidly to awfulness.[30] We can entertain options that will allow us to avoid future pain, or we can withstand immediate pain for longer-term benefit. We can evaluate long-term plans and their possible consequences. How this is achieved is a topic of ongoing research, but is not well understood.[31] What we do know is that deferring gratification typically involves consciousness and the engagement of the imagination as future effects are considered, but may also be mediated by long-established habits, ingrained by the reward system.[32] Such evaluation should not, however, be construed as "strictly cognitive," in the sense of being uninfluenced by emotions, as perhaps calculating the sum of 29 and 57 would be. In fact, evaluation of envisaged future events, a constraint satisfaction process, is shaped by signals from the valencing circuitry that is the very core of being, being well, and being social. "Cool" reason is not devoid of emotions. Rather, it is balanced by attitude-emotions such as prudence, vigilance, and caution.

There is yet another evolutionary modification to the mammalian brain, which involves the vagus nerve and the brainstem (figure 3.7). The *vagus nerve* is a kind of conduit for detailed signals to and from all aspects of the body—internal, muscular, skeletal, and skin. In mammals, a new branch of the vagus developed that modified in a profound way a specialized behavioral response to danger—namely, freezing. Freezing can confuse a predator, who likely relies on motion to know where exactly the prey is. A lizard may freeze when startled, for example. Neuroscientist Stephen Porges[33] suggests that the mammalian modification of the freezing circuitry permits a new behavior that keeps the stillness but drops the fear, thus allowing for *immobility without fear*.

Why is that important? Because mother mammals need to be immobile without fear, while remaining vigilant. From the perspective of reptiles, this is an odd combination of states, but to suckle infants for hours and hours of her day, a mother mammal needs to lie fairly

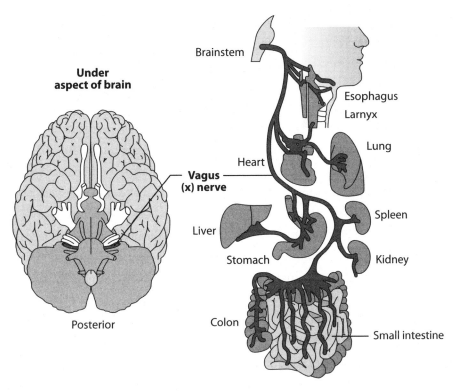

Figure 3.7. The vagus nerve pathways. Left: Schematic diagram showing the location of the vagus nerve (tenth cranial nerve) as it enters the brainstem, as viewed from the underside of the brain. Right: Schematic showing the exceptionally broad range of innervation by the vagus nerve. "Gut feelings" are believed to rely on signals from the vagus nerve. Copyright Bloomsbury Educational Ltd., www.clinicalexams.co.uk/cranial-nerves-system.asp; adapted with permission.

still so the infants can feed on their only food. Her body must not be in shut-down mode, but ready to respond to threats and intruders. When mammalian mothers are still, the body and brain must not respond as though freezing *with* fear, for freezing with fear would mobilize the sympathetic system, damping the effects of oxytocin, and hence interrupting the flow of milk. Instead, the lactating mother must be still, while calm and relaxed, and ready if danger arises. The female mammal also needs to be somewhat still for copulation (consider the heifers that basically stand motionless while the bull energetically deposits sperm), and for birth (where dashing around would be dangerous to mother and child). So the vagus nerve, which is frequently taught as just another boring old cranial nerve to be memorized for the anatomy test, is, in mammals, a very special part of our social nature.

For rats, mice, and many other mammals with a small prefrontal cortex (PFC) relative to body size, the brainstem and other subcortical structures are the principal players in integrating signals and making decisions, such as whether to flee now and feed later, whether to fight on or try again another day, whether to incur pain to defend the young against a predator. In primates, such as monkeys, chimpanzees, and humans, the larger prefrontal cortex means that the subcortical structures participate in but do not usually dominate the decision-making, though during panic, they may.[34] Hence in primates there is a more flexible, and more complex, connection between stimuli and behavior. Barry Keverne has described this looseness as a kind of liberation from fixed action patterns seen in small-brained mammals.[35]

The excursion into the briar patch of pain, fear, pleasure, and the reward system has one more payoff. Prediction, as neuroscientist Rodolfo Llinás points out, is the ultimate and most pervasive of brain functions.[36] That is because in guiding behavior, predictive operations serve survival and well-being. The better the prediction, the more likely the individual is to survive predation, find good food, and avoid perils. Like the magic of compound interest, predictive capacities become exponentially more powerful and abstract with the expansion of neural networks between sensory input and motor output. Early mammals could use their neocortex to anticipate more effectively when a circumstance might end in trouble. Large-brained mammals can be even more clever in their predictions and behavior.[37] For social mammals, anticipating what others will do is supremely valuable: will another share, bite, hit, mate, or what?

Anticipations of social trouble normally carry emotional valence, and motivate preventive action in some form suitable to the circumstance. Moreover, the infant learns to anticipate the mother's behavior, and that of its littermates, coming to predict what is likely to follow certain preparatory movements—play, hurting, and so on. This, suggest Don Tucker and colleagues, marks the modest beginning of inner representation of the goals of other individuals,[38] a representation that is more abstract than a prediction of movement, but dependent on learned associations mediated by neocortical neurons.[39] Only recently have animal behavior experiments been aimed at discovering whether nonhuman animals have a mental model of others' goals and point of view, and some of the results are surprising. A scrub jay, as ethologist Nicola Clayton has shown, does understand what other jays can see, and tailors its caching behavior accordingly.[40] If a high-ranking jay can see another jay's nut cache, the caching jay moves it; not so if the watching jay is low-ranking.

Chimpanzees have been shown to be entirely capable of adjusting their behavior in a comparable way. Consider the mother chimpanzee who anticipates that her young chimp will provoke a hostile reaction in the alpha male if he were to make a grab for the adult male's food. The mother feels anticipatory pain seeing the juvenile's purposes, and whisks him off before the trouble starts. In humans, these humble but useful predictive tools lead to a more full-blown schema of others' mental states, namely, a "theory of mind," full of abstract representations such as "goals" and "beliefs." (The neurobiology of "theory of mind" will be discussed more fully in chapter 4 and 6.)

Increased neurobiological understanding of attachment in mammals fits with the observation that the nervous system is highly conserved across species: neurons are much the same and function in much the same way in humans and mice and slugs; the palette of neurochemicals affecting neurons and muscles is substantially the same across vertebrates and invertebrates; the basic pattern of body and brain development is similar across vertebrates and invertebrates. The striking thing is that modest modifications in existing neural structures—an expansion of an auditory area, or a magnification of a region representing touch on the fingers, for example—can lead to new outcomes, such as a much greater ability to discriminate sounds patterns or touch patterns.[41] Along these lines, neurobiologist Jaak Panksepp suggests that the distress at social separation seen in mammals may be a modification of a more ancient *place preference*—with concomitant anxiety in alien places—regularly seen in nonmammals.[42] Familiarity is pleasant because it allows for greater predictability, and that means a reduction of anxiety. The pleasure of being among others in the group exploits the circuitry for feeling comfortable in safe and familiar, "rest and digest" conditions. The evolutionary changes in mammals whereby distress is felt at separation from those to whom we are attached are perhaps modest modifications from the point of view of brain circuitry, yet they yield something quite new at the macro level: extending caring to others.

Biological evolution does not achieve adaptations by designing a whole new mechanism from scratch, but modifies what is already in place, little bit by little bit. Social emotions, values, and behavior are not the result of a wholly new engineering plan, but rather, an adaptation of existing arrangements and mechanisms that are intimately linked with the self-preserving circuitry for fighting, freezing, and flight, on the one hand, and for rest and digest, on the other. The pain of exclusion, separation, and disapproval, for example, does not require a whole new system, but exploits, expands, and modifies what is already in place for physical pain and homeostatic emotions in pre-mammalian species. In the next section we take a closer look at how some mammalian nervous systems expanded attachment beyond the tight circle of offspring.

Mate Attachment

Though sometimes assumed to be a uniquely human pattern, long-term mate attachment is found in about 3% of mammals, including beavers, marmosets, titi monkeys, gibbons, the California deer mouse, prairie voles, and pine voles.[43] Most mammals, however, even if they are social, are either promiscuous or seasonal in their mating. A far higher proportion of bird species—around 90%—have strong mate-preference and long-term bonding.[44] Our closest living relatives—chimpanzees and bonobos—are not long-term pair bonders, and the same goes for most rodents and monkeys.

Long-term mate attachment is a highly significant form of sociality: we love the other, we want to mate with him, be with her, to see her prosper, care for him. We feel distress at separation or when our partner is hurt or threatened. When a partner dies, the survivor is often depressed and sometimes fares poorly.[45] Mate attachment does not, however, imply sexual exclusivity, as genetic studies on rodents and humans reveal.[46] This may have something to do with genetic diversity, and studies on the common mole rat, with the evocative scientific name *Cryptomys hottentotus hottentotus*, do suggest this.[47] But the question now is this: when we see strong mate preference in prairie voles, for example, what in the brain explains why a prairie vole is inclined to bond with its mate for life, but a montane vole is not?

Voles are rodents that look rather like chubby mice with short tails. Prairie voles and montane voles, though physically resembling, are quite different in their sociality: prairie voles mate for life; montane voles display no partner preference. Male prairie voles guard the female and the nest against intruders, and males share parenting of the pups, licking, retrieving, and defending them. In montane voles, only females rear the pups, and then for a briefer period than prairie voles. General levels of sociability are also distinct. Placed randomly in a large room, prairie voles tend to cluster in fairly chummy proximity; montane voles are content to be loners.

Prairie vole male-female pairs provide the basis for extended family groups, with siblings helping out with the younger pups. Not so for montane voles. Because the montane and prairie voles are very similar in the gross structure of their brains, they can be compared at the microstructural level to discover what neurobiological differences might explain these striking differences in sociality.

In the 1970s, Sue Carter, a neuroendocrinologist at University of Illinois, had been studying the effects of hormones on brain and behavior when she observed that prairie voles formed strong mate preferences, and moreover that the bond forms with the first mating. Wondering about this striking phenomenon, she suspected that sex hormones—probably estrogen—held the key to explaining the voles' unusual attachment patterns. While it was a good guess, her experiments did not support the estrogen hypothesis. Looking elsewhere for answers, she pondered biologist Barry Keverne's remarkable neuroendocrinological work on sheep.[48] Keverne's lab had shown that injection of the neuropeptide oxytocin into the brain of a sexually naïve ewe could bring on full maternal behavior, including ewe-lamb bonding As any sheep farmer knows only too well, getting a ewe to bond to an orphan lamb is very difficult to achieve, even for ewes who have just delivered a stillborn lamb and would be ready to tend a lamb. So the effect was very striking indeed. If mother-offspring attachment is mediated by oxytocin, could mate-bonding be an extension of that? Carter's hunch turned out to be very fruitful indeed, and it set in motion a huge range of research. Learning about this research, I began to suspect that this was the link to the kind of caring that we associate with human moral behavior.[49] This, perhaps, Hume might accept as the germ of "moral sentiment."

The Mechanisms of Mate Attachment

As mentioned, oxytocin is a very simple, very ancient, peptide; it is a chain composed of nine amino acid links (hemoglobin, for contrast, is a hugely complex chain, with more than five hundred amino acid links). OXT has a sibling molecule, *arginine vasopressin* (AVP), and they appear to have evolved from a common ancestor, differing in only two amino acids. Like OXT, AVP is found in the brain as well as the body, where it plays a crucial role in maintaining blood pressure and water balance.

OXT and AVP are naturally released in the hypothalamus, and diffuse quite widely to other subcortical areas, such as those involved in reward (including the nucleus accumbens), in regulation of sexual behavior (the septum), and in regulation of parenting. OXT is more abundant in females than in males. AVP is released from other subcortical areas, including the medial amygdala, the lateral septum, and the periventricular nucleus, and is more abundant in males than in females. The levels of AVP increase as the male enters puberty, and it is released during sexual arousal, falling just before ejaculation. In male rats, OXT promotes erectile function, peaking during orgasm, and falling to baseline levels about thirty minutes after orgasm.[50] *Corticotrophin releasing factor* (CRF) is also a highly important player in mammalian social life. It is associated with stress, and hence with anxiety and its discomforts. When animals feel safe and comfortable, their OXT levels rise and their CRF levels decrease from a "fight or flight" level. Correspondingly, anxiety is reduced. Notably, however, moderate levels of CRF increase bonding in male prairie voles.[51]

To exert their effects, OXT and AVP bind to specific receptor-proteins on the surface of neurons, and hence the role of OXT in behavior depends on its relative abundance, but also on the density of receptors on neurons in a particular brain area. For example, female rats showing higher levels of licking and grooming of their infants have a greater density of OXT receptors than other females. OXT has only one kind of receptor, but AVP has two different receptors in the nervous system. Binding to one plays a role in mate bonding and parental behavior, whereas binding to the other is associated with anxiety and aggression, typically in mate guarding.[52]

In the research *so far*, the main neurobiological contrast between male montane voles and male prairie voles is that the latter have a much higher density of receptors for AVP and OXT in *two very specific* subcortical regions of the brain: the *ventral pallidum* and the *nucleus accumbens* (both part of the reward-and-punishment system; see figure 3.8).[53] Although all mammals have both OXT and AVP in the central nervous system and all have receptors for both, experiments have shown that it is the receptor density in these two specific and highly interconnected regions that marks a key difference in social behavior. If the receptors are experimentally blocked so that the OXT or AVP cannot bind, then the treated voles do not bond after the first mating, and do not exhibit the social behavior typical of prairie voles. Neurobiology being what it is, we should not be surprised if further factors, such as variations in neural circuitry and in levels of other hormones, play an important role in whether individuals in a species typically form long-term bonds or not. Hence the facts about high receptor densities correlating with long-term bonding are best thought of as the beginning of the story, not its end.

What exactly is the effect on neurons when these two peptides, OXT and AVP, bind to their respective receptors? Investigation of these details is underway; complete answers are not known. Moreover, the answers are certainly going to be complex, even in voles, since the neurons affected are part of a wider system, meaning that what is going on elsewhere—in perception, memory, and so forth—will have an impact. At the risk of simplification, we can note some properties that do stand out. OXT is released during positive social interactions, and has been shown to inhibit defensive behaviors, such as fighting, fleeing, and freezing. It appears to do so by interacting with the hypothalamic-pituitary-adrenal axis to inhibit activity in the amygdala, an evolutionarily old structure whose various functions include the regulation of fear responses. OXT release also tends to downregulate (dampen) fight-and-flight autonomic responses in the brainstem, and in general reduces the nervous system's reactivity to stressors. Significantly, its effects are context-sensitive. OXT administered to male rats increases aggression toward an intruder but decreases aggression toward pups.

Does the profile of receptor density seen in prairie voles extend to other monogamous species? It appears that the answer is *yes* for

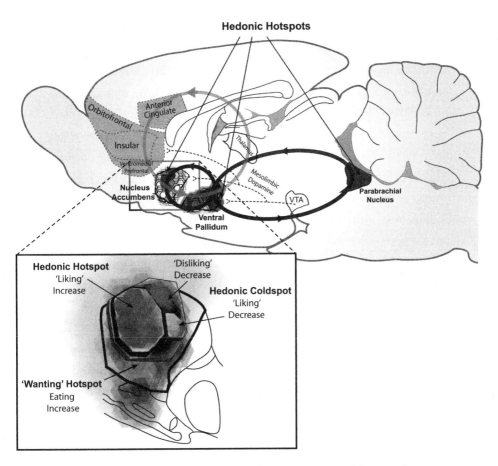

Figure 3.8. Drawing of a rat brain, showing the main circuitry of the reward system. Three crucial subcortical structures are the nucleus accumbens, the ventral pallidum, and the parabrachial nucleus. The main cortical structures connected to the hedonic hotspots are the anterior cingulate, the orbitofrontal cortex, the insula, and the ventromedial frontal cortex. The VTA (ventral tegmental area) contains neurons that release dopamine, and these neurons project into the ventral pallidum, the nucleus accumbens, and the orbitofrontal cortex, and are important in reward learning. All the structures and pathways exist also in the human brain. From Kent C. Berridge and Morten Kringelbach, "Affective Neuroscience of Pleasure: Reward in Humans and Animals," *Psychopharmacology* 199 (2008):457–80. With permission.

marmoset monkeys,[54] titi monkeys,[55] and the California deer mouse (*Peromyscus californicus*). By contrast, promiscuous species such as the rhesus monkey and the white-footed mouse, *Peromyscus leucopus*, have an OXT and AVP receptor profile similar to that of the montane (promiscuous) vole. The comparable facts concerning receptor density in human anatomy are not yet determined, since injection methods to tag the receptors cannot be done in living humans, and are not effective when performed on dead brains. Nevertheless, because mechanisms and structures are highly conserved across species, a reasonable guess is that those humans who do form long-term, stable relationships will have receptor densities that are more like that of the prairie voles, marmosets, and gibbons than like that of montane voles and chimpanzees.

Investigating human gene-brain-behavior links, Heike Tost recently reported that a particular variant of the gene for the OXT receptor (OXTR) correlates with some types of variability in sociality seen in humans, including some types of social impairment.[56] The *allele* (the OXTR gene is known as rs53576, the allele as rs53576A) is correlated with specific anatomical differences (relative to normal controls): decreases in gray matter size in the hypothalamus; increased connectivity between hypothalamus and amygdala and between hypothalamus and anterior cingulate cortex; and in males only, an increase in gray matter volume of the amygdala.[57] In testing whether this made any difference to brain activity during an emotionally salient task, they found decreases in the level of amygdala activity.

Behaviorally, the allele was associated with decreased sociality (the urge to belong, empathy for others, sensitive parenting, the capacity for long-term attachments, and so forth) using well-established self-rating scales.[58] No techniques yet exist to determine directly the receptor density and distribution in live subjects, hence the focus on neural structures known to sequester OXT (e.g., the hypothalamus) or to be richly connected to areas that have OXT receptors (for example, the amygdala). To explain the variation in social temperament, Tost et al.

suggest that in those carrying the rs53576A allele, the nonstandard structure and connectivity between the hypothalamus, amygdala, and anterior cingulate may typically generate less positive or even negative feelings about social interactions. What a control subject might find a mildly pleasurable interaction, such as chatting with a stranger in a grocery store queue or helping a neighbor pick up dropped groceries, these subjects find unpleasant. This is plausible, given what is known about the important role of the amygdala in feelings of fear and fear responses, and also in positive social responses.[59] Many factors play a role in sociality in humans, and as we shall discuss in chapter 5, single genes seldom have big effects, but are part of multinode gene-networks, and part of gene-brain-environment networks with recurrent loops. Accordingly, the finding regarding one significant variant of the gene for OXTR, while important, is likely to be only a part of the story of human sociality and its variability.

To get a feel for these other factors, consider that there is a generational effect of maternal behavior on the infant's OXT levels, and on its subsequent social behavior. Michael Meany and his colleagues showed that mother rats that have high levels of maternal behavior also have high levels of OXT; the recipients of their maternal behavior also have high levels of OXT that was shown to be causally related to the mother's licking and grooming. When those female pups mature and have their own litters, they too are highly maternal, and have high OXT levels, and their babies in turn have high levels of OXT.[60] Cross-fostering tests show that the parental behavior in early experience of the infants is more influential in this outcome than genes.[61] A similar result has now been shown in rhesus monkeys.[62] In humans, higher OXT levels correlate with high levels of maternal interactions, which in turn correlate with high levels of OXT in the babies. As Ruth Feldman and her colleagues suggest, there is a biofeedback loop between OXT, parenting, and infant social competence in nonhumans, and this may obtain in humans as well.[63]

What Else besides Oxytocin?

More is known about the role of vasopressin in males than in females. In males, it is essential for bonding to a mate, and probably also plays a role in aggression, especially in defense of juveniles and the mate. Nevertheless, in some conditions AVP has effects opposite to those of OXT. Thus administering AVP to a male vole increases his level of activity and arousal, and is more associated with defensive postures than with "friendly" postures. Whereas OXT administration to females reduces mobility and induces quietness, AVP administered to males seems to have the contrary effect. The OXT and AVP systems of course interact with other hormones such as estrogen and progesterone, both prenatally and after birth. They interact as well with neurotransmitters such as dopamine and serotonin,[64] and the details are under study. (Neurotransmitters, of which there are many, are substances secreted by one neuron, then binding to another after diffusing across the space between the two neurons, thus constituting a form of communication between spatially separate neurons. The released substance will increase or decrease the probability that the receiving neuron will be activated.)

In addition to the OXT and AVP systems, the *dopamine* system appears to be important to the expression of social behavior. Dopamine is a neurotransmitter that plays multiple roles in many functions. It has two receptor types, D1 and D2,[65] that are particularly relevant to social behavior, and each has distinct functionality. Dopamine is known to be crucial in learning, and mediates neuronal changes in the reward/ punishment system as animals learn about the world and come to predict one event from the occurrence of another. For prairies voles to attach to their mates, for example, they need to be able to recognize which vole they mated with, and recognition requires learning, and learning requires dopamine.

Dopamine has recently been identified as having a role both in pair-bonding and parenting behavior. Access to D2 dopamine receptors is necessary for formation of a pair-bond, while activation of D1 dopamine receptors blocks pair-bond. Following formation of the bond, D1 receptors are upregulated, preventing formation of a second bond. In order for dopamine to function in pair-bonding, its D2 receptors have to be located next to the OXT receptors on the same neurons in the reward system; for females that co-localizing arrangement must exist in the nucleus accumbens, while for males, it must exist in the ventral pallidum (both structures being part of the reward-and-punishment systems).

Release of the endogenous opiates follows the reunion of separated animals or the satisfactory response to distress calls from the juveniles.[66] Behaviorally, this can be observed in the joy displayed by one dog when reunited with his pal or his master, a behavior that is completely distinct from the subdued look of sadness when the suitcases appear in the hall. Reunited dogs, for example, will lick each other on the face, jump to each other, wag energetically. The precise nature of the role of the endogenous opiates, and their interactions with other hormones such as prolactin, and with OXT and AVP, remains to be worked out. While the story is incomplete and becomes more complex the more we know, the core of the story—that receptor density for OXT and AVP is associated with attachment—draws some of the mystery out.

I have emphasized that there is a complex relationship between OXT and CRF, a stress hormone, but one of the most remarkable findings expands the complexity into the unexpected realm of general health and wound healing. Stressful conditions, such as being in a restraint, can slow down wound healing, a result shown in both humans and rodents. Importantly, administration of OXT has been shown to speed up wound healing in stressed rats. This finding raises a very intriguing question concerning the relationships between OXT and other substances known to play a role in wound healing, such as circulating *cytokines* (part of the immune system response), and other substances that reduce inflammation. In a recent paper, neuroscientist Jean-Philippe Gouin and colleagues[67] tested wound healing in human subjects. Thirty-seven couples, displaying varying degrees of affection or tension, were admitted for a hospital visit for 24 hours, during which they participated in a "structured social support interaction task." OXT and AVP levels in saliva were measured upon entry. One finding was that higher OXT and AVP levels were associated with supportive, affectionate human relationships, lower levels with "negative communication" in couples. For the "wound," everyone received a small suction blister on the forearm. The progress of the blister's healing was evaluated every day for eight days, and then again on the twelfth day. The basic finding, statistics aside, was that individuals with high OXT levels showed significantly faster healing, and women with high AVP levels did also.

Also noteworthy here are proposals to use oxytocin for therapeutic purposes in treating cases of posttraumatic stress disorder (PTSD) that are resistant to cognitive therapy. Because of the relationship between levels of oxytocin and feelings of safety, trust, and pleasure in the company of others, and because weakening conditioned fear responses involves weakening the amygdala's reactions to a stimulus, the therapeutic strategy is under serious consideration.[68]

Male Parenting

The forgoing traces some of what is known about pair-bonding, but a little more needs to be said about the mechanisms whereby male voles show spontaneous parental behavior. New data suggest that this too is mediated principally, but not exclusively, by OXT and AVP. Neuroscientist Karen Bales showed that reproductively naïve male voles spontaneously engage in *alloparenting* (rearing of non-kin) of pups to which they are exposed, showing both passive parenting (huddling over the pups) and active parenting (retrieval and licking).[69] If, however, the males are treated with substances that block the OXT receptors and the AVP receptors, alloparenting is reduced and attacks on pups are increased. At lower doses of the blockers, the response to pups is slower, and attacks are fewer, suggesting dose dependency. If only one receptor type (either OXTR or AVPR) is blocked, there is no effect. So either receptor seems to be sufficient for mediating the alloparenting. Finally, it turns out that in a reproductively naïve male prairie vole, mere exposure to pups increases his level of OXT, lowers his level of corticosterone (a stress hormone), and enhances the probability of later bonding with a female.

Evolutionary biologists may ask why male prairie voles bother with parenting, let alone alloparenting—what is in it for them and their genes? After all, the montane vole pups do well without their fathers helping out. So far as I know, there is no entirely settled answer. The environments of montane and prairie voles are rather different, however, and the prairie voles are probably more vulnerable to predation by hawks and kestrels than montane voles, who usually have ample protective cover among rocks and bushes in the woods. On open prairie, males' parenting can help defend the nest, and by bringing extra food, males can raise stronger pups that are more resistant to predation. In any case, the fact that OXT- and AVP-mediated parenting behavior is seen in males also suggests a more general idea, namely that in mammals, expanding sociability may be achieved by rather minor genetic modifications, resulting in modifications to the circuitry, neurochemicals, and receptors to support new levels of sociability.

Early on in the research on monogamous pair-bonding in prairie voles it was suggested that the genetic differences between monogamous pair-bonders and others might be linked to variants in a particular stretch of DNA that regulates expression of the vasopressin receptor. That particular stretch of DNA was discovered to be longer in prairie voles than in montane voles, thus raising the question of whether this might be true of other species in which mates form long-term bonds. Further research on other species has challenged that suggestion, alas. Multiple mechanisms are clearly involved, and genetic analysis shows that monogamous mating patterns have evolved multiple times in mammals, and at least twice even within the genus *Peromyscus*.[70] Talk of a "gene for monogamy" is muddled.[71]

What about *human* mate attachment? Are we, by nature, like prairie voles? The answer seems to be that humans are flexible in their mating arrangements. Strong attachments are certainly common, but according to anthropologists George Murdock and Suzanne Wilson, 83% of societies allow polygynous patterns of marriage. Depending on conditions, however, even if polygyny is allowed, most men are of modest means and hence are likely to have only one wife.[72] Consequently, *de facto* monogamy may prevail, though the wealthier men may have more than one wife. In historical times, it has been well documented that a wealthy man may have a special, long-term attachment to one particular female, even while enjoying, and perhaps impregnating, various other women. So even when polygyny is the local practice, individual inclination may result in long-term attachments.

In the other 17% of societies, both modern and ancient (e.g., Greece and Rome), monogamy has been the practice. The explanation for the cultural variation of marriage practices probably rests mainly with variation in ecological and cultural conditions, and in particular, with whether there are conventions for heritability of property and other forms of wealth, along with wealth to be inherited.

Drawing on historical and ethnographic data, evolutionary biologists Laura Fortunato and Marco Archetti argue that when there are multiple wives each with children and hence multiple heirs, transferring resources to all heirs results in a depletion of their fitness value; for example, the patches of land to bequeath get smaller and smaller, and less able to support the families that depend on the land.[73] A man might select one particular wife whose children inherit all the wealth, but this makes for competition among offspring, and is generally an unstable solution. In these conditions, a more stable strategy for enhancing the well-being of one's own offspring would be to have one wife, be sure of the paternity of the offspring, and invest heavily in the welfare only of her children. Fortunato and Archetti note that monogamy emerged in Eurasia as agriculture became widespread, with land and herds as an important source of wealth that could be passed to heirs. Once certain practices become the norm, once they are seen to bring benefits and to circumvent troubles, once they are reinforced by social approval and disapproval, they do of course seem to reflect the only right way for things to be.

What Is the Connection between Attachment and Morality?

The probability is that OXT and AVP and a spectrum of receptor distributions are important elements in the explanation of human styles of sociability, and this neurobiological understanding has broader implications for the origin and basis of human morality. Humans, like baboons, marmosets, wolves, and some other mammals, are intensely social. Our brains are structured to see to our own interests, but also to those of kin and kith. Though social life brings many benefits, it does increase within-group competition, and rivalry for resources between siblings, mates, and neighbors. Social problem-solving, grounded by attachments, but also shaped by concern for reputation and by fear of punishment and exclusion, leads to ways of reducing conflicts, such as those involving external threats and internal rivalries. Thus in humans, monogamy as a social practice may be a good solution to reducing competition for females, and for bequeathing resources. Some social solutions are more effective than others, allowing for stability and security within the group, but others may be socially unstable in the long run or may become unsuitable to the well-being of members when conditions change. Social behavior and moral behavior appear to be part of the same spectrum of actions, where those actions we consider "moral" involve more serious outcomes than do merely social actions such as bringing a gift to a new mother. That social and moral behavior are part of a single continuum is modestly supported by neuroscientific data showing that whether a subject sees a merely social event or a conventionally "moral" event, the same regions of the prefrontal cortex show increased activity.[74]

In humans, cultural practices, conventions, and institutions steadily change as solutions to social problems become entrenched. Practices may be picked up explicitly, as in learning not to lick your knife at table, or implicitly, as in learning the acceptable forms of hugging and kissing with kith and kin. Humans are learners *extraordinaire*, and imitators *plus extraordinaire*. Sometimes without much awareness, we pick up mannerisms, styles, technologies, practices, and in-group symbolism.

Social problem-solving is probably an instance of problem-solving more generally, and it draws upon the capacity, prodigious in many humans, to envision and evaluate the consequences of a planned action. It also draws upon the capacity, probably connected to playfulness, to modify current practices and technologies as conditions change. Cultural variability in social practices of humans is well documented by social scientists, and covers a broad span, from land ownership to banking regulations to appropriate responses to insults to suitable forms of humor.[75] But just as there are common themes across cultures in body decoration or animal husbandry, so there are common themes regarding punishment, conflict resolution, mate and child interactions, property ownership, and group defense. Shunning as a form of punishment for social misbehavior, for example, is common across many cultures and species, and reconciliation following conflict typically involves touching and stroking, and often a ritualized submissive posture. Shunning and reconciliation touching are each linked to distinct changes in the neural circuitry that causally implicate distress or comfort, respectively.

The commonality in social practices is owed in part to similarity in our basic social desires and their neurobiological mechanisms, conserved across all mammals but with distinct modifications in distinct species.

Exactly what about the human brain allows for cultural accumulation, and what ecological conditions support it, remains unsettled.[76]

In chapter 4, we shall look more closely at what we can learn from neuroscience and anthropology about extending trust and cooperation beyond small groups of kin-related individuals, to acquaintances, and then to strangers.

• • •

In mammals, many brain processes participate in sociality, but three major factors stand out: (1) urges to care about the welfare of self, offspring, mates, and affiliates; (2) the capacity to evaluate and predict what oneself and others will feel, and do, in particular circumstances; and (3) a neural reward-and-punishment system linked to internalizing social practices and applying them suitably—more generally, linked to learning the expectations and ways of parent, siblings, and other group members.[77]

The form that sociability takes in individuals of a species depends on their niche and on how they make their living. Sociability is not all-or-nothing, but comes in degrees. Cougars tend to be minimally social, humans tend to be intensely social, and ravens are somewhere in between. Sociability can also depend greatly on food resources. As Benjamin Kilham has shown in his wonderful studies, black bears, standardly classified as solitary creatures save for mother-cubs groups, will be surprisingly social so long as there is lots of food to feed everyone.[78] Lastly, within a species there is considerable variation among individuals, and as noted above, some of this may depend to some extent on genes for the receptor of OXT, but also on infant-parent interactions. Some humans are highly group-directed and reputation-sensitive, while others live contentedly on the fringes of society, happy in their eccentricity; at the extreme, there are humans with distinctly disadvantageous social impairments, such as autism.

If moral values are anchored by the neurobiology of sociability, and if cooperation is an important morally relevant behavior, the next step in our investigation is to look more closely at cooperation, and finally to inquire how it is that trusting, cooperative interactions can regularly occur between unrelated friends and strangers. At the same time, we need to be aware that there is a dark side to sociality, and in humans, it can be very dark indeed.

4. Cooperating and Trusting

The extension of caring to dependent infants, and then to mates, kin, and affiliates, marks the crucial shift that makes us social.[1] At the center of the intricate web of neural connections is oxytocin (OXT), a powerful peptide that in mammals has been recruited in organizing the brain to extend self-care to infants, and thence to a wider circle of caring relationships. Oxytocin has been associated with trust, owing largely to its role in raising the threshold for tolerance of others, and to its down-regulation of fear and avoidance responses. In conditions of safety, when the animal is among friends and family and the OXT levels are higher, there is mutual grooming, touching, and general relaxation. Additionally, grooming and touching appear to raise levels of OXT, relaxing one further, indicating a biobehavioral loop.[2] Although the relationship between OXT and the endogenous opiates is not well understood, from the little that is known, it appears that in many conditions where OXT is released, endogenous opiates are also released. Doing good feels good — at least sometimes.

The aim in this chapter is to look more closely at *cooperation* as a social phenomenon, and how it might be related to social behaviors that depend on OXT, AVP, and their portfolio of receptors. A preliminary point, to be defended and illustrated below, is that there is unlikely to be one lone mechanism for mammalian cooperation. A second preliminary point is that some social behaviors in some species, such as alloparenting (parenting of others' babies) by male prairie voles, may not be selected for as such, but may be a situation-dependent by-product of the circuitry needed to support a behavior that *is* selected for, such as a general disposition to care for pups, which typically gets deployed when the pups in the vicinity are in fact one's own. Third, as Robert Boyd and Peter Richerson argue,[3] in humans, the extension of cooperation beyond kin and known tribal members was likely common only after the advent of agriculture, about 10,000 years ago. When the main source of food was hunting and foraging, as for example among the various Inuit tribes when anthropologist Franz Boas studied them in 1883–84, competition for resources tended to keep groups separated, save for annual gathering for barter of tools and other goods, and for reconnecting with family.[4]

New data from field anthropologists studying the patterns of behavior in people from widely different communities as they play money-exchange games such as Ultimatum and Dictator (discussed later in this chapter), strongly suggests that levels of trust and cooperation with strangers are greater among those whose groups have greater "market integration" (a term used by anthropologists to mean the proportion of calories in their diet that are purchased or traded, as opposed to being grown or hunted by the groups themselves).[5] As human settlements grew in size to thousands of individuals, the advantages of interacting with non-kin familiars and with strangers may well have become clear enough to stabilize practices of fairness in trade. Incrementally, institutions arose to structure cooperation and punish noncooperation—institutions regulating activities such as land ownership, inheritance, bartering and trade, and sharing the cost of common services.[6] Both simulation models and anthropological data show that larger groups tend to have more tools, and more complex tools, than smaller groups.[7] Analogously, larger groups tend to have more complex social practices, including those for trade and exchange that involve trust.

Trust can be expanded beyond the circle of kin and familiar folks if the institutional arrangements can be counted on to assure a reasonable level of trustworthiness of participants, known and unknown. While the character of nascent institutions was shaped by background social attachments to kin, it was likely also affected by assorted other factors: the nature of the problems that needed to be solved, the willingness to punish violators, the idiosyncrasies of the individual players, and the history of earlier ways of doing things. Cooperative systems that extend beyond the small group of kin and familiars are thus likely to be highly dependent on culture—on the beliefs, and attitudes, and learned habits that are widely adopted in a community, and on the institutional arrangements for reducing the risk of cooperating with strangers.

A shared religious institution may, as Joseph Henrich and colleagues note, be one way of extending the boundaries of trust to ephemeral interactions with strangers.[8] This effect is probably owed to an increment in predictability of behavior when conventions are known to be shared. Market-integrated individuals are more likely to show trust in dealings with strangers than are hunter-gatherers who have not experienced the benefits of cooperative conventions, and have not acquired the habits suitable to such interactions. When established institutions become unreliable or corrupt, trust is withdrawn, with suspicion of strangers, familiars, and even family members becoming the standard. In recent times, a stunning and tragic example of this breakdown in institutional trust occurred in the former Soviet Union under Stalin and thereafter.[9]

What Exactly Is Cooperation in Mammals?

Cooperation is not a single pattern of behavior, as, for example, suckling is. What counts as cooperation in animal behavior? For clarity, evolutionary biologists give precise meaning to *cooperation* and other associated terms:[10]

1. A behavior is *social* if it has fitness consequences for both the actor and the recipient.
2. A behavior that is beneficial to the actor and costly to the recipient (+/–) is *selfish*.
3. A behavior beneficial to both is mutually *beneficial* (+/+).
4. A behavior that is beneficial to the recipient but costs the actor is *altruistic* (–/+).
5. A behavior that is costly to both actor and recipient is *spiteful* (–/–).
6. Whether a behavior is *costly* or *beneficial* is defined on the basis of
    (i) the lifetime fitness consequences (not just the short-term consequences)
    (ii) the fitness consequences relative to the whole population, not just relative to the individuals or social group with which the individual interacts.
7. *Cooperation* is a behavior that provides a benefit to another individual (recipient) and whose evolution is dependent on the beneficial effect for the recipient.

These clarifications are very useful, especially in elucidating what "fitness consequences" involve, since evaluations of fitness of a behavior are apt to be a source of disagreement among scientists, some of which turn out to be merely semantic. Despite the usefulness of these definitions, I have misgivings about adopting the last one, concerning cooperation, for the purposes of this book, as it seems to exclude quite a lot of behavior in humans that normally gets called *cooperative*. Here is why.

To count as cooperation, according to the definition above, the behavior must be *selected for* because of its beneficial effects on the recipient. Thus shared parenting is probably selected for in marmosets and titi monkeys, as is sentry behavior in meerkats. The rationale for the clause is this: without the "selected for" clause, one could say that elephants cooperate with dung beetles to provide dung aplenty. But nobody really thinks that elephant bowel movements ought to count as cooperation with dung beetles. Rather, the dung beetle evolved to take advantage of a rich food source, which, as it happens, is copiously available where there are elephants. So to forestall absurdity of that kind, write into the definition the requirement that the behavior considered cooperative was selected for its beneficial effects on the recipient. The elephants' copious evacuations were not selected for as part of the interaction with dung beetles, hence they are not an instance of cooperation.

While the amendment serves to rule out the elephant-and-dung-beetle case as cooperation, it runs the risk of ruling out perfectly ordinary cases of human cooperation. When my neighbor and I engage in a joint tractor-repairing effort because it is advantageous for both of us and extremely difficult to achieve singly, this would commonly be called cooperation. Nevertheless, because joint tractor-repairing behavior presumably is not the outcome of natural selection (our brains did not evolve to repair tractors), then by the biologist's definition, our venture does not qualify as cooperation. It does, nevertheless, count as mutualism (+/+), and by the biologists' definition, this term does not imply that the behavior has been selected for (see the definition above). If we abide by the definition of cooperation as it is offered, we must live with the consequence that most human joint ventures fail to be cases of cooperation. When evolutionary biologists are talking only to other evolutionary biologists, this may be fine. The trouble in this context is that the definition requires common usage to change, often a recipe for rampant confusion unless the conversational benefits are overwhelming. We could use *mutualism*, but that word does not have all the forms that *cooperate* does: I can say "Should we cooperate?" but it sounds silly to say "Should we mutualize?" "Billy is not cooperative at school" would come out as "Billy is poor at mutualism" or some such.

The definition may be too restrictive also for some forms of primate cooperation (in the loose sense). Field anthropologists at the Lomas

Barbudal Biological Reserve in Costa Rica observed white-faced capuchin monkeys cooperating to retrieve a juvenile monkey from the coils of a boa constrictor. Some groupmates physically attacked the snake, while others worked to extract the monkey from the snake's coils. When the alpha male arrived on the scene, he began hitting, and possibly biting, the snake from the opposite side that the mother attacked. This was effective in rescuing the juvenile. Capuchins also cooperate in aggressive attacks on other capuchin troops.[11] Because capuchin groups tend to be very close knit, it may be that freeing a groupmate from a snake is not selected for as such, but strong caring is. Thus they cooperate in diverse circumstances, and depending on the groupmate's dilemma, they will act appropriately, using their past knowledge and problem-solving capacities.

Under "cooperation," here is what the Oxford English Dictionary lists as a primary meaning: "the action of co-operating, *i.e.* of working together towards the same end, purpose, or effect; joint operation." The idea of "a joint effort" seems to capture many collective human endeavors, and possibly those of other primates as well. And it does seem to exclude the elephant and dung beetle case. The advantage of this description for our purposes here is that it leaves open the questions of selection, requiring merely some level of goal-directedness. This may not serve so well for ant and fish behavior, but perhaps for our purposes temporarily conforming with the OED might be wisest, recognizing that no single definition of cooperation may be suitable for all species.

Cooperation in Mammals: A Few Examples

Cooperation in mammals can take many forms, from grooming others so as to remove parasites, as baboons and chimpanzees do, to forming an ever-shrinking circle so as to corral fish, as dolphins and orcas do.

Some species engage in "territorial chorusing," in which individuals collectively produce alarm calls in response to possible intruders into the territory. Within a species, cooperative behavior is sensitive to local conditions and to individual variation in sociality.

Grooming appears to give pleasure to both parties, likely because the circuitry supporting licking infants and being licked—crucial to cleanliness as well as to normal brain development—has a hedonic aspect that persists into maturity.[12] Although considerable efforts have been made to explain the grooming of others in terms of selective advantages to this social arrangement, a simpler explanation for at least some grooming behavior may just be that it feels pleasurable for both the groomer and the groomed, and if there is not much else to do anyhow, this is a pleasant way to spend time. The cost is minimal, and the reward is significant. The human predilections to hang around chatting has strong similarities to grooming in baboons.[13]

Huddling together for warmth is also a form of cooperation, albeit a simple one, where all in the huddle benefit from tolerating close proximity on a wintry night. Huddling is a typical form of parent-offspring behavior, and adults huddling against the cold is an obvious solution to a weather problem. Hence this is not a case where explanation invoking specialized circuitry or particular genetic contributions is needed. Notice that according to the biological definition of *cooperation* in the list in the previous section, if it is just a solution to a problem the brain figures out, huddling together in the cold may not qualify as cooperation, but only as mutualism.

Cooperative hunting, seen in wolves, African wild dogs, dolphins, orcas, and birds such as ravens, is a very different form of cooperation from huddling together, not least because it involves sophisticated, organized, and fast responses to changing contingencies.[14] The neurobiology of cooperative hunting is difficult to study, and not well understood. But the mammals who do it tend to be smart, in some everyday sense of the word, and they may also be adept at predicting others' behavior based on attributions of goals and intentions. Nevertheless, references to intelligence raise difficulties regarding how intelligence is defined, measured, and tested in nonlinguistic animals, not to mention issues concerning the significance of field observations versus tests in captivity, and the ever-handy rebuke of "anthropomorphism."[15]

Alloparenting is believed to be rare among mammals, but it does occur. Although studies of captive chimpanzees have suggested they are indifferent to the plight of non-kin, a recent report by Christophe Boesch and colleagues of field studies revealed eighteen cases of orphan adoption, half by males.[16] In prairie voles the males engage in parenting, but the siblings also typically help with the pups. Alloparenting is also seen meerkats, where an auntie or two helps the mother tend the pups, and, in the course of tending, may even begin to lactate. Wild red ruffed lemurs engage in extensive alloparenting, including infant stashing in the tree canopy, nest guarding, transporting, and allonursing.[17] Common marmosets, living in large groups, also show alloparenting, including carrying and provisioning, especially by siblings.

Actively rejecting others' offspring may be selected for in those mammalian species where the young can walk immediately after birth, and could readily poach on another mother's resources if not deterred. Sheep, for example, discourage needy orphans (recognized by smell) by kicking them or head-butting them away. That alloparenting is rare among sheep is not surprising, owing to the cost of juvenile care, and the low level of benefits that can be expected in return. Nevertheless, the fitness consequences of alloparenting (across the whole population, and in the long run) appear to be positive for some species, depending on how they make their living.

There can also be interspecies cooperation (mutualism again), as when ravens lead coyotes to an elk carcass, in the expectation of doing the cleanup job once the basic butchering has been achieved by the sharp teeth of the coyotes.[18] Humans and dogs, of course, have cooperated in many ways, possibly for as long as 30,000 years.[19] Baboons have been used by humans to help herd goats. Hoesch provides details on how a female baboon, Ahla, led the farmer's goats out in the morning, gave alarm calls if she spotted a predator, brought the goats back to the barn in the evening, groomed the goats, and regularly escorted separated juvenile goats back to their mothers.[20]

Trust and Oxytocin: What Do We Know about Its Effects on Humans?

The main hypothesis of this book, that morality originates in the neurobiology of attachment and bonding, depends on the idea that the oxytocin-vasopressin network in mammals can be modified to allow care to be extended to others beyond one's litter of juveniles, and that, given that network as a backdrop, learning and problem-solving are recruited to managing one's social life. One might predict, therefore, that cooperation and trust are sensitive to OXT levels. This raises an important question: can changes in OXT levels affect human cooperative behavior?

One line of research aims to explore the effects of OXT on human behavior by administering measured amounts of OXT and seeing whether trusting or cooperating behavior changes. OXT is usually administered using a nasal spray, so that the OXT reaches the subcortical brain via the pathways from the odor receptors in the nose to the olfactory bulb in the brain. The next step—finding a suitable behavior on which to get measurable, meaningful effects—requires nontrivial ingenuity.

Michael Kosfeld, a neuroeconomist (he studies how decisions are made by the brain), asked this question: if subjects were given OXT before playing an economic game where trust played a decisive role in success (i.e., earning more), would they be more successful than the control subjects not given OXT?[21] To answer this, he and his colleagues selected the decision-making ("economic") game "Trust." Here is how Trust works. One player is the *investor*, one the *trustee*, but they cannot talk to or see each other and their identities are masked. This is artificial, of course, but it avoids confounding factors such as friendships and appearance that could influence behavior. Each player is given $12 (real money) to begin. The investor can then invest either $0, $4, $8, or $12 with the trustee. The amount invested is tripled by the experimenter and paid to the trustee; for example, if the investor invests $8, the trustee accumulates $(8 \times 3) + 12 = 36$. The trustee can send back however much, or little, he wishes to the investor. The more the trustee sends back, the more the investor will be able to invest in subsequent rounds of the game, and hence the better the two will do in the long run. Simple math reveals that earnings of both are maximized if the trustee, after receiving a first investment, signals trustworthiness to the investor by returning a goodly proportion. Under these conditions, if the investor then trusts and invests generously, the dyad can earn quite a lot over the course of several rounds. The question is whether the investor's level of trust can be modified by administering OXT.

The answer is *yes*. Subjects in Kosfeld's experiment played four rounds. Those who were given OXT in a nasal spray were significantly more willing to trust the trustee, sending money 45% of the time (versus 21% in controls given a placebo spray) and sending an average of 17% more money per transfer than controls. Importantly, the effect disappeared if the investor believed he was playing with a computer-program trustee rather than a human. Furthermore, though it had an effect on *investor* behavior, OXT nasal spray had no effect on *trustee* behavior. This makes sense because success in the trustee role does not require trust, though, as we see below, the trustee does need to recognize when an investor is sending a signal of trust (i.e., investing a large amount of his pot).

Can specific psychiatric conditions affect the capacity for trustees and investors to successfully negotiate cooperative behavior? Suggestive evidence comes from studies of individuals with *borderline personality disorder* (BPD). BPD is a serious mental illness characterized by instability in moods, interpersonal relationships, self-image, and behavior, and also by low levels of trust or randomly fluctuating trust.

It is believed to afflict about 2% of the population, and causes great hardship to family members as well to as the individual with BPD.

Neuropsychologist Brooks King-Casas studied fifty-five subjects previously identified as suffering from BPD, in order to identify brain regions related to the pathology.[22] In the behavioral part of the study, BPD subjects played the role of trustee in the Trust game for ten rounds, while a healthy control played the role of investor. The comparison class was composed of investor-trustee dyads made up of healthy control individuals. As noted earlier, the best strategy for maximizing income is for the investor to start with a fairly high investment, and for the trustee to send back more than the investor sent forward as a signal of trust (recall that the experimenter triples the amount the investor sends to the trustee). Once trust is established, the prudent investor sends more to the trustee. If trust is ruptured by a shortfall, generosity by the trustee signals a willingness to repair the rupture.

BPD trustees were poor in setting up or maintaining a trusting relationship, and poor in signaling trustworthiness to repair a trust rupture, even when urged by the experimenter to do so. As a result, the BPD subjects' profits were lower in the game than those of healthy volunteers. They also self-reported lower levels of trust than did healthy controls. Using fMRI imaging, cortical activity levels of healthy controls and BPD subjects were compared. One difference involved the anterior insula, known to play a role in the generalized discomfort of rejection and norm violation (see chapter 2). More specifically, King-Casas found that in BPD subjects, receiving an "unfair" small amount from the investor evoked no increase in activity in the anterior insula, while *sending* an unfair amount did. This suggests that these subjects expected to be treated unfairly, while at the same time being capable of evaluating what an unfair amount was. By contrast, in healthy controls, "unfair" transactions, either received by them or sent by them, were accompanied by anterior insular activity increase. King-Casas suggests that the effect in the anterior insula is consistent with the typical BPD profile of low expectation of others and negative evaluation of others.

An obvious experimental idea is to administer OXT to BPD subjects, and see whether trusting behavior and the capacity to recognize trust-me signals are improved. While a simple idea in the abstract, this is actually a heroically difficult experiment in reality, given the number of patients that would be needed to get statistically meaningful results, along with their disinclination to participate, owing to their BPD. Nevertheless, the existing results from the King-Casas study do give an intriguing glimpse into the complexity of trust, and remind us that a diminished capacity to form and maintain trusting bonds with others forestalls the many benefits of cooperation. Individuals who have difficulty forming trusting relationships are at a huge disadvantage.

In a recent study, using healthy male subjects, neuropsychologist Carsten De Dreu explored a question of particular interest to my hypothesis: what effect does intranasal OXT have on in-group cooperation, cooperation with out-group members, and hostility to out-group members?[23] As with earlier studies, the test involved playing a game with real money where a subject could benefit relative to his in-group fellows (two others), the whole group could benefit, or a loss of money could be inflicted on the out-group with minimal cost. As structured, cooperation maximizes group benefits, selfishness maximizes personal benefits, and spite allows punishment of the out-group with no costs to in-group members, but costs the out-group members. Here is the setup: Each subject was given €10. Each euro kept was worth €1 for the individual; for each euro contributed to the *within-group* pool the experimenter added €0.50 to each in-group member, including the contributor; for each euro contributed to the *between-group* pool, the experimenter added €0.50 to each in-group member, including the contributor, and, also, *subtracted €0.50 from each out-group member*. This arrangement allows for expression of hostility to members of the out-group, essentially at no cost to members of the in-group. Men were assigned to groups randomly, and the game was played on a computer, with players' contributions kept confidential from one another.

The basic finding was that the men who got the intranasal OXT treatment were significantly more cooperative (on average gave more to the in-group than did controls), but out-group hostility remained much the same. Classing subjects as *egoists* (usually kept their allotment), *in-group cooperators* (usually contributed to the in-group pool), or *out-group haters* (usually chose the spiteful contribution), these numbers were found: in the control group, 52% *were egoists*, 20% were in-group cooperators, and 28% were out-group haters. By contrast, for those getting intranasal OXT, 17% *were egoists*, 58% were in-group cooperators, and 25% (not significantly different from controls) were out-group haters. This result does suggest a major effect of OXT on cooperation within the group. The artificiality of the setup is of course what allows for quantifiable results, but it does mean that it is essential to display caution in generalizing to conditions of normal, everyday life, where individuals often know each other well, have past interactions that affect their feelings, and belong to a range of groups that sometimes overlap and sometimes do not (family, coworkers, golf partners, yoga mates, church members, etc.) Incidentally, it is puzzling that about a quarter of subjects, both those with intranasal OXT and controls, were willing to inflict cost on members of the out-group, individuals who, apart from the experiment, had no connection to the subjects.

In a different study, using intranasal OXT administered to healthy controls, neuroeconomist Paul Zak sought to determine whether there might be any differences between levels of generosity in a situation where the recipient can respond and can thereby affect the final outcome, versus a situation where the recipient takes what is given but cannot react.[24] Each pair of subjects played either the "Ultimatum" game or the "Dictator" game, once only. In Ultimatum, decision-maker 1 (DM1) is given a sum of money, say $10, and he can offer a portion (anything between $0 and $10) to decision-maker 2 (DM2). If DM2 accepts the offer, they both pocket what they have, and the game is over. If DM2 *rejects* the offer, however, *neither gets anything*. Tests using Ultimatum show that on average American subjects tend to consider as insulting offers below some minimal amount, say 30%, and when offered such an amount, will reject the offer, thus punishing both players.

In Dictator, the recipient makes no decisions, provides no response, and hence cannot affect the final outcome. The money is simply split as the dictator specifies. Thus there are two players: dictator-donor and passive recipient.

How does the behavior of OXT donors compare with that of controls? In Ultimatum, the OXT donors offered 21% more than the controls. In Dictator, however, there was no effect of OXT. This implies that the anticipated reaction of the recipient (DM2) player in Ultimatum, with the possibility of rejection of the offer and loss, was a factor in the decision regarding what to offer. Zak interpreted the results as showing that the OXT subjects playing Ultimatum have a greater feeling of empathy for the recipients who might be offended by a very low offer and hence reject it. I suggest a slightly different explanation: that a greater sense of awareness of the other's feelings exists in the OXT subjects, as they anticipate the interaction. A stingy offer could be rejected, and none of us likes the feeling of an offer rejected, as it signals disapproval. On this interpretation, OXT subjects are a little more sensitive to rejection than controls, and hence a little more alert to the feelings and likely responses of the other player. This interpretation raises the broader question of mental attribution, and more generally, of predicting of behavior in a social context by making use of "theory of mind."

Success in the social world depends on learning the ways and profiles of others; the more sophisticated and accurate the predictive machinery—modeling the mental states of others—the greater the advantages. It seems probable that in mammals, elaboration on the rudimentary capacity to detect and respond to distinct types of distress in offspring gave rise to fancier capacities to attribute goals, intentions, and emotions to others, as larger brains made it possible to anticipate future events, including the social behaviors of others, that might be punishing or rewarding.[25] Chapter 6, on social skills, will look more closely at hypotheses concerning the neural basis for mental attribution. Here we only consider whether changes in OXT levels can affect accuracy in "theory of mind" tasks. The answer is *yes*. In studying the role of OXT in identification of others' psychological states, psychologists showed that male humans given intranasal OXT improved their performance on the task. They used the "Reading the Mind with the Eyes" test, first developed by Simon Baron-Cohen.[26] In the test, the subject sees a person expressing an emotion, but only the *eyes* are visible. The subject's task is to choose, from four options, what the person is thinking or feeling. The first few examples are easy, but the examples get more difficult as the test progresses. The improvement with OXT was most pronounced for the most difficult examples.

Just when we think we have a phenomenon more or less nailed, new data show that everything is vastly more subtle. It turns out that administration of OXT via nasal spray has different neural effects in men than in women, performing a task requiring recognition of emotional faces. Thus one study used fMRI to scan male subjects while they observed either fearful faces and scenes, or neutral objects. Consistent with earlier data showing that OXT reduces levels of fear and anxiety, they found decreased activity in the amygdala and in the brainstem areas to which it connects in subjects who had received OXT spray.[27] However, a later study by another group of researchers found different results in this experiment when the subjects were women.[28] More exactly, their OXT subjects (relative to controls) showed *increased* activity in the left amygdala, the fusiform gyrus, and the superior temporal gyrus in reaction to observations of fearful faces. In all these areas, plus the inferior frontal gyrus, activity was increased during observation of angry and happy faces (see figures 3.6 and 6.3).

In a study involving the administration of AVP to men and women subjects, psychologists found remarkable differences between the sexes in their facial responses and perceptions when shown unfamiliar faces.[29] Women given AVP responded to pictures of unfamiliar *women* with affiliative (let's-be-friends) facial expressions, and saw the faces as more friendly than female control subjects. Men given AVP responded to pictures of unfamiliar men with activity in the corrugator (frown) muscles of the forehead, and perceived the faces as more unfriendly than normal control subjects. The researchers noted that in all subjects, threatening and fearful faces increased the autonomic response, and hence increased anxiety levels. The data, they suggest, support the hypothesis that when anxious, the women are disposed to use a "tend-and-befriend" strategy, not a "fight-or-flight" strategy, which may be more typical of men.[30]

Sex differences will likely turn out to be increasingly important in this unfolding research,[31] given the sex differences in densities of receptors for AVP (more in males than females) and OXT (more in females than males), and to differences in subcortical circuitry in structures such as the hypothalamus.[32] Of course, within sexes there is also individual variability.

Are subjects given intranasal OXT aware of any shifts in their conscious attitudes, such as feeling more trusting? So far the answer seems to be *no*. The effects appear to be subtle, below the level of conscious awareness, though further studies may find a more noticeable effect on awareness in some situations. Many people ask whether the effects of OXT are sufficiently positive that we should spray it around when we wish to reduce tensions, say during a debate in the UN General Assembly. Various companies advertise OXT nasal spray on the Internet as a way of improving trust in business affairs.[33] We need to exercise great caution in delivering OXT. Sometimes we tend to suppose that more of a good thing is an even better thing (as Mae West famously said, too much of a good thing is wonderful), but often that is not so. Biology, as is well known, often conforms to the ∩ curve—the maximally effective range for something is often neither the maximum nor the minimum. Too much of a good thing can be catastrophic.

Curious about the effects of extra OXT, neuroscientists were surprised to observe that administering additional OXT in an otherwise normal female prairie vole results in a *weakening* of attachment to her mate. Moreover, extra OXT may also cause a female prairie vole to go into estrus.[34] While OXT may well have quite different effects in human females, these data are a cautionary reminder that OXT is a powerful hormone that plays many roles in the brain and body. One would no more casually play around with OXT than one would with the sex hormones estrogen or testosterone. The fact is, no one has the slightest idea of the long-term effects of OXT medication, and children may be especially vulnerable.[35]

Another warning is provided by a result obtained by Thomas Baumgartner and his colleagues. Control subjects playing Trust typically adjust levels of money transactions when a breach of trust occurs—when a stingy amount is passed back from the trustee. Subjects given OXT, however, tend to continue with their high level of trust, regardless of the breach.[36] In a realistic situation, that persistence is unlikely to serve a subject well. In real life, persistent trust in the face of countervailing evidence might be like the ever-generous fool who is repeatedly hoodwinked by the con artist. We teach children to be wary of certain kinds of behavior and certain sorts of people; willy-nilly trust is a recipe for disaster.

Can OXT be used therapeutically? Some research groups have asked whether in autism spectrum disorder (ASD) the circuitry for feeling safe and trusting, and the related capacity for reading of emotions, is somehow amiss, and whether the condition might be improved by administering OXT. Given the difficulty of finding any effective treatment for ASD, this has seemed like an appealing line of investigation. With this in mind, neuroscientist Eric Hollander intravenously administered OXT to a group of autistic and Asperger's adults, and then asked them to detect the affect (happy, indifferent, angry, or sad) in the speech they listened to. To avoid confounding variables that would make interpretation impossible, the content of each sentence was neutral: only the *prosody*—the rhythm and intonation—had emotion. Compared with control subjects, the test group showed significant improvement with the administration of

OXT, and the improvement was retained over a period of weeks.[37] In a related experiment, the researchers noted in OXT subjects a decrease in the repetitive behavior characteristic of ASD. In a more recent set of experiments, neuroscientist Angela Sirigu reported significant positive effects after OXT inhalation in thirty high-function subjects with ASD.[38] These effects included longer eye contact, and stronger interactions with socially cooperative computer partners in the computer game Cyberball. Suggestive as these results are, the data need to be complemented by further studies, and it is important not to overinterpret the results.

If there is an OXT component to ASD, then what specifically in the OXT network might be altered—for example, OXT receptors or pathways within the subcortical structures, or OXT synthesis in the hypothalamus? Or something else yet again? Several studies reported variations in the gene (i.e., polymorphisms) for the OXT receptor based on genetic analyses of families with members affected with ASD. Unfortunately, more recent analyses have cast doubt on the hypothesis that the OXT receptor, or its abnormalities, play a major role in ASD.[39] Exactly why the experimental administration of OXT has the reported effects remains unclear.

One other result, described as very preliminary, has shown that levels of OXT in the cerebrospinal fluid of women who had suffered childhood abuse or neglect were significantly lower than those who had not.[40] Categories of abuse included physical abuse, emotional abuse, sexual abuse, and physical or emotional neglect. Subjects who had reported trauma in more than three categories had OXT levels much lower than those who had trauma in only one. Nothing about their social behavior was reported, and the authors warn that a larger sample should be studied, and that nothing could be concluded regarding causation. Still, if further research provides evidence that there is a causal connection, then this result will have important social implications. As mentioned in chapter 3, another possible therapeutic intervention concerns post-traumatic stress disorder that is resistant to cognitive therapy. While a medical intervention is an important direction to explore, here too, caution is the watchword.[41]

Although the data discussed show that there are important relationships between social behavior and OXT, AVP, and their receptors, understanding the precise nature of those relationships will require understanding much more about how decisions are made, as well as how perception affects and is affected by emotions.[42] Withal, bear in mind that OXT should not be dubbed *the* sociality/cognitive function molecule. It is part of a complex, flexible, interactive network of genes, gene-neuron-neurochemical-environment interactions, and neuron-body interactions.

Punishment and Cooperativity[43]

Benefits accrue to social animals who cooperate, but even more benefits can accrue to cheaters who avoid paying the costs. Without selective punishment, cheaters would likely be more successful in spreading their genes, and would over time come to dominate the population.[44] Since they have not, the fair assumption is that cheating is deterred. Shunning is one powerful form of punishment in highly social mammals, especially because a loner likely has access to fewer resources and is vulnerable to more predators. For example, over a seven-year period, Bekoff found that 60% of yearling coyotes trying to make it on their own died, whereas only 20% of yearlings living in the group died.[45] Punishment for failing to play fair has been seen in coyotes, and punishment in rhesus monkeys for failing to call out after finding a good feeding site has been observed.[46]

As biologist Tim Clutton-Brock remarks, the problem of free-riding (taking the benefits but paying no costs) may be attenuated when, as is typical, the group is small, individuals in a group know each other well, and cooperation usually involves no time delay between the cooperative costs and receipt of benefits.[47] Under these conditions, there may be little opportunity for free-riding to evolve. Early hominin life likely satisfied these fairly simple conditions. In addition, of course, many individuals in a group are likely to be related, and hence OXT-mediated "caring" would be extended to kin.

The issue of punishment of the stingy and the shirker has been studied in humans using economic games. In one experiment, neuroeconomists Ernst Fehr and Simon Gächter compared participants' behavior in a public goods game,[48] which works this way: each player is given a pot of money, and can put any amount in a public coffer, or hold some back for himself. The experimenter multiplies by some factor, say 3 (greater than 1, but less than the number of players), the amount in the public coffer, and for the final payout, the money in the public coffer is split evenly among the players and each keeps whatever amount he held back in his own pot. The group as a whole does best when everyone puts all their money in the public coffer, and that is pretty obvious to players once the rules are explained. An individual subject, however, can do best if everyone else puts their money in the public coffer and he holds all his back. This is because his return on every unit of money he himself puts into the public coffer is less than one.

Fehr and Gächter had subjects play in two conditions: one with punishment and one without. Importantly, punishment in these experiments was costly for the individual doing the punishing; a player had to pay a fee using his own pot in order to punish another player by reducing that player's private pot. The game was played in groups of four individuals, and in order to prevent the development of individual reputation over the course of the ten rounds of the game, subjects were anonymous and the composition of the groups randomly changed from round to round.

Fehr and Gächter found, in line with previous studies not incorporating punishment, that in the non-punishment condition, contributions to the public coffer were moderate initially and decreased in subsequent rounds until free-riding (zero contribution) was the dominant strategy. In sessions in which punishment was available, they found that subjects were willing to punish other individuals who contributed little or nothing to the public fund. Subjects did this even though they incurred a cost by doing so and despite the fact that, due to the randomized, anonymous-players design of the game, they might not interact with the punished individual again (and would not know it even if they did).

The availability of punishment had a dramatic effect on cooperation: average contributions were two to four times higher in the punishment condition than in the non-punishment condition, with contributions in the final rounds being 6 to 7.5 times higher when punishment was available. Moreover, even the mere possibility of punishment was effective as a means of increasing cooperation. In one experimental session, subjects played a twenty-round game in which punishment was not available for the first ten rounds; here, the standard pattern of contributions decreasing from an initial modest level was observed. But when punishment became available in round 11, contributions immediately jumped to almost four times their round 10 level and continued increasing through the twentieth and final round.

A later study by Fehr and Gächter suggests that the relevant psychological mechanism of so-called "altruistic punishment" is negative emotion directed toward non-contributors (defectors).[49] (The punishment is "altruistic" because, as noted above, it is costly and does not yield any material benefit to the punisher. It turns out that people will pay a cost to punish defectors even when they are "third parties," individuals who are merely observing an economic game rather than playing in it themselves.[50]) The design and behavioral results of this study were very similar to those of the previous study. Participants played a randomized public goods game in punishment and non-punishment conditions, where players were anonymous. Contributions were once again significantly higher in the punishment condition, and the mere switch from punishment to non-punishment or vice versa resulted in an immediate change in average contribution levels. When the option of punishment became available, contributions immediately jumped and continued to increase; when it was removed, contributions immediately dropped and continued to decrease. Once more, the frequency of punishment was high despite its costliness: in a typical six-round game, 84.3% of subjects punished someone at least once, and 34.4% punished more than five times. Defectors were by far the most frequent targets of acts of punishment, receiving 74.2% of the total, and cooperators (those who contributed above-average amounts) tended to be the ones doing the punishing.

In this last experiment, Fehr and Gächter hypothesized that negative emotions toward defectors might be the proximate mechanism behind altruistic punishment. To test this, they presented subjects who had just finished playing the public goods games with written descriptions of hypothetical scenarios. A sample scenario might be as follows: "Let's say you decide to invest 16 francs in the project. A second member invests 14, a third invests 18, and a fourth invests 2 francs. You now accidentally meet this fourth member. Please indicate your feelings toward this person."[51]

Subjects indicated how much anger, if any, they would feel using a seven-point scale, with seven representing the highest level of anger. In the version of the scenario reprinted above, in which the individual had contributed a high amount relative to the defector, 47% selected an anger level of six or seven, and a further 37% selected an anger level of five. Moreover, when subjects were instead presented with a hypothetical scenario in which they were the defector (and the other individuals were high contributors) and asked to rate how angry they expected the others would be, they again gave very high anger ratings, with 74.5% choosing six or seven, and a further 22.5% choosing five.

These studies suggest that anger is a powerful driver of a canonical moral behavior, namely, the punishing of wrongdoers. Moreover, most people are aware of this, as indicated by their ratings of the anger they would expect others to feel toward them if they defected. This latter fact may help explain the immediate jump in contributions observed upon the switch from non-punishment to punishment conditions.

Accordingly, the emotions probably have an important role not only in the actual process of making moral judgments but also in motivating behavioral responses to these judgments and, through the anticipation of such emotion-driven responses, in deterring people from behaving immorally in the first place.[52]

Not surprisingly, reputation turns out to be important in emerging patterns of cooperation and punishment in public goods games, much as in real life.[53] Neuroeconomists Bettina Rockenbach and Manfred Milinksi were interested in how building a reputation as stingy (my description) can be used by non-stingy players in punishing the stingy by withholding help. Additionally, they wanted to compare the effectiveness of withholding help on the basis of reputation, with costly punishment, where the punisher has to pay to punish the stingy. Once again, the public goods game, described above, was the experimental tool. The idea was that reputation could be rewarded or punished in the post-game period (really, the second stage of the public goods game).[54] The options were *no punishment, costly punishment* (it costs a punisher to punisher a free-rider), and what they called *indirect reciprocity*, a post-game transaction which requires some explanation: After the public goods game has been played a number of rounds, three monetary units are made available to players who have built "good reputations" in the public goods stage. They have the opportunity to help another player, who, in turn, then gets the donation tripled by the experimenter. Indirect reciprocity presents the opportunity of less costly punishment, namely refusing to help a free-rider. Some experiments were run where both kinds of punishments, indirect reciprocity and costly direct punishment, were an option. Free-riders could be hit twice by a punisher—once as a direct cost, and once as a refusal to help. Games with the two-punishment profile turned out to be especially interesting.

At the risk of oversimplifying this very complex experiment, the basic finding of interest here is that although subjects initially tend to choose the no-punishment group, most, when give the choice, switch their preference to the group *with* the costly punishment option, and prefer the dual punishment system to the single (direct only). Further, when the less costly punishment is available, two things happen: instances of costly (direct) punishment—as measured by the average number of punishment points doled out per member of the group—drop by about half, but when direct punishment is used, it is more severe than when it is the only option available.[55] (I note, for what it is worth, that this would be my inclination as a player, on grounds that if someone freeloads even while aware of the dual punishments at hand, then he may play more generously henceforth if he gets a strong nudge.) Finally, there is a net increase in contributions to the public-good pot, thus increasing everyone's take. These experiments also serve as a reminder that punishment can take many forms, that there can be interactive effects, and that people are willing to exact a cost to freeloading, even when it involves a cost to themselves. A reputation for trustworthiness is a value.[56]

The Effect of Social Tension on Cooperativity

Against the background appreciation of the evolutionary changes to mammalian brains that extend caring beyond the self, we can examine the suggestion that in highly social animals, the level and degree of cooperative behavior may be enhanced or enabled by temperamental differences typical in a species, where those temperamental differences are themselves related to the social structures typical of groups in the species. The neurobiology of the relevant temperamental differences is in its infancy; here we will simply focus on the behaviors themselves.

Depending on the species and the conditions, social life can have a lot of background tension. Group living provides benefits, but it is bound to create within-group rivalries, competitions, and irritations. Individuals may live together, and forage together, but lower-ranking individuals are wary of more dominant individuals in feeding, getting good sleeping spots, and copulating; the more dominant have to be wary of challenges from the upstarts. When tight hierarchical organization prevails, and aggression is used to maintain respect or to advance in rank, then fear of those lower, or higher, is more or less constant.

For males, the main benefit of high rank is access to females, and preferential access to food; the obvious cost is associated with maintaining high levels of vigilance and intermittently putting the challengers down in physical interactions. A less obvious cost concerns the limitations on cooperation for mutual benefits, owing to the difficulty of establishing cooperative arrangements across ranks. To illustrate, a high-ranking male tends to be intolerant of sharing food with a lower-ranked male, who in turn sees no advantage in cooperating with a higher-ranked male who can be expected to monopolize the proceeds of cooperation. This suggests that cooperation may be rather limited in those social organizations where dominance hierarchies are strong and maintained by aggression. Cooperation among females may also be sensitive to rank, as it is in baboons. Research on the question of social tension and its effect on cooperation has been undertaken by psychologist Brian Hare,[57] and I will outline the main results below.[58]

Bonobos tend to be more easygoing than chimpanzees, arguably because their foraging territory south of the Congo River is much richer in large fruiting trees than the chimpanzee territories north of the Congo River.[59] As Hare explains, "Overall, large patches of fruit and higher levels of high quality herbs to fall back on when fruit is unavailable reduce the costs of co-feeding and group living for bonobos relative to chimpanzees."[60] With reduced foraging competition, there is likely to be reduced aggression, and hence a more relaxed way of life. Being more relaxed means that bonobos will be tolerant of the close presence of others during eating. Chimpanzees, by contrast, have a rather high-stress social organization with a tight male dominance hierarchy. Bonobo females within a group bond closely, especially along kin lines, and although males have a dominance hierarchy, a coalition of females can gang up on a male. A female bonobo will take food from a male, and bite one who resists, a behavior rarely seen in chimpanzees though also common in ringtail lemurs. Chimps are also less likely than bonobos to tolerate the close presence of down-rank or up-rank bystanders during feeding.[61]

Hare wondered whether easygoing bonobos might be more successful than the more socially tense chimpanzees in solving a problem that requires cooperation of two animals.[62] To test this, they trained the chimps by putting two food dishes separated by 2.7 meters on a platform in a cage. To retrieve the food, the two animals had to simultaneous pull on the attached rope-ends. The chimps easily learned the task, whereupon the experiment changed, and only a single dish of food was placed on the platform, which the chimps could share if they successfully pulled the platform forward. What Hare observed was that if a chimpanzee could work with a "friend" (roughly, a chimp of the same rank), cooperation was smooth, but if he or she was paired with a nonfriend, such as a more dominant chimp, cooperation failed, even though both knew what they needed to do to get the food. In other experiments, a chimp was allowed to go and get another chimp to help in the one-dish food-pulling task. Under this condition, chimps generally picked someone both friendly to them, and known to be skilled at the task.

How did the bonobos do? Even though the chimps were given more experience at the task, the naïve bonobos outperformed them. This was clearly evident when only one of the food dishes was baited, and after pulling the platform in, the two bonobos shared. Chimps were wary of the one-dish situation, either to avoid interacting with a more dominant chimp, or because the more dominant chimp could not suppress entitlement to all the food. Interestingly, comparable results had been found earlier for two species of macaques—the strict-hierarchy rhesus, known to be socially prickly, were less cooperative than the loose-hierarchy tonkean, known to be more socially easygoing.[63]

In analyzing their results, Hare suggests that a relatively high level of cooperativity in a species may be enabled by the social system and the temperamental portfolio that supports it. Both chimps and bonobos are clever enough to know how to cooperate, and to understand the value of a cooperative interaction. But cooperation is much more constrained by the chimpanzee social system. As noted, in the wild bonobos live in a richer resource environment than chimpanzees, which may have allowed the more easygoing temperament to flourish. Arguably, the chimps' higher levels of aggression and social intolerance during feeding may in general have served them fairly well in a highly competitive food environment.

Evolution and Human Cooperation

Reliable cooperativity may, as Hare suggests,[64] emerge most easily in primates when individuals have easygoing temperaments. This raises an interesting question: temperamentally, are *Homo sapiens* more like chimps or bonobos? Was life as a savannah ape easier and more prosperous than life in the forest, and if so, did that permit a relaxed social organization that was conducive to lower tension and more cooperation? Temperament in humans seems highly variable, stretching from the tense and edgy to the laid-back and lackadaisical, and is doubtless influenced by many environmental factors. Nevertheless, the capacity of contemporary humans to tolerate and enjoy the company of diverse others suggests that in some respects, we may, on average, be temperamentally a little more like the bonobos than like chimpanzees. Against this supposition is the sobering fact that aggression toward individuals in the out-group appears to be easily triggered when conditions favor it, and such aggression has been a standard feature of human life in historical times.[65] In any case, a temperament more easygoing than that of chimpanzees, and entailing less fear and aggression within the group, may have permitted cooperation to occur regularly enough that cooperation came to be a standard practice, valued for its results.

Anthropologists suggest there is a link between the evolution of the human disposition to engage in cooperative behavior on the one hand, and the lengthy period of dependency of human juveniles, and the need for kin—mates, and often siblings and friends—to help to rear the young, on the other. Cooperative parenting, according to this hypothesis, is a successful reproductive strategy.[66] Cooperation of the parents may be even more fundamental. Since human infants require exceptionally long periods to mature, it behooves fathers to play a big role in seeing their offspring to a successful independence. Mating with many females and fathering oodles of offspring that compete poorly is, given the dependency of human juveniles, a less successful strategy in spreading one's genes than helping to rear a selected few to competitive strength. Assuming that cooperative parenting increases fitness, long-term pair-bonding might, other things being equal, be a better reproductive strategy than promiscuity. Sarah Hrdy discusses several Amazonian hunter-horticultural tribes (including the Ache, Canela, Mundurucu, and Mehinaku) in which women routinely consort with more than one man, who then cooperate in rearing "their" children. As she notes, "the Ache believe that fetuses are a composite from several different men with whom the mother had sexual relations. . . . The Mehinaku joke about this joint paternity, referring to it as an 'all-male collective labor project.'" These children have a better survival rate than those without several fathers.[67]

Hrdy suggests that cooperative parenting may reach back at least to *Homo erectus*, whose brain capacity (800–1100 cc^3) was about twice large as that of the australopithecines, though smaller than *Homo sapiens*. Her argument is twofold. First, brain size predicts that the juveniles would have had a long period of dependence, thus favoring cooperative parenting (the head has to be small enough so that the baby can pass through the birth canal, and expansion of the head and the brain can occur after birth). Human babies are exceptionally immature at birth, in contrast, for example, to rhesus monkeys. Hrdy's second point concerns sexual dimorphism. Fossils indicate that in *Homo erectus*, males were only about 18% larger than females, roughly similar to the sexual dimorphism in modern humans (males are on average

about 15% larger than females), but very different from existing chimpanzees and the australopithecines. The relevant biology here is that
polygamous species—including birds and mammals—tend to be more
sexually dimorphic in size than monogamous species, presumably so
that males can police the harem and fend off other suitors. Thus male
gorillas are huge relative to female gorillas, male elephants seals are
huge relative to the females. But in the marmosets and titi monkeys,
who are monogamous, males and females are indistinguishable in size.

Mate attachment is believed to bear on sexual dimorphism in the
following way: with less need to fight to keep a harem secure and in
line, a male's massive size becomes a cost rather than a benefit. Aside
from keeping themselves fed, human males need to help provide the
female with rich food to feed the fetus or keep the milk flowing, and
the slow-developing juveniles need a high-quality diet to mature.[68] Unless a massive size serves some other purpose such as fighting other
males, it can end up just being a big mouth to feed. Over generations,
when the mates bond for the long term, the large size differences between males and females tend on average to disappear. Another factor,
suggested by psychiatrist Randolph Nesse,[69] is that up to a point, male
generosity and cooperativity might function rather like the peacock's
tail. That is, if a male can display generosity and cooperativity, this reflects well on his overall strength and health, and hence his desirability
to females as a mate. On Nesse's hypothesis, then, some social virtues
are favored by sexual selection.

Cooperative parenting, in tandem with stable pair-bonding anchored by an oxytocin and vasopressin network, might mean that
for hominins, for example, *Homo erectus, Homo heidelbergensis,* and
Homo sapiens, trust was a typical baseline within the family, and
could readily be extended to kin and affiliates in a small group, benefits and reputation permitting. Trust permits cooperation, and cooperation is associated with richer food resources, especially in beating
off competing scavengers and in hunting large animals. Aggression
within the group is modulated, while aggression toward the out-group

might remain high. Like chimps, humans do kill individuals in the out-groups, and unlike bonobos, female dominance over males seems moderately rare.[70]

Data from marmoset behavior provides modest support for the hypothesis that cooperative parenting accompanies, and eases the way for, more comprehensive cooperation. Marmosets form long-term pair-bonds and share parenting, and turn out to be somewhat similar to humans in being willing to act so as to help another, without any expectation of reciprocity or reward. Neuroeconomist Ernst Fehr's lab set up the experiment so that one caged marmoset could pull a tray to enable a marmoset visible in an adjoining cage to get a piece of food, though the puller still could not get to the food. The kindly marmosets reliably put out the effort to help a stranger (all the appropriate controls were in place) even when they could see that they themselves had nothing to gain, and the lucky marmoset was, though visible, not a friend or family member.[71] Chimpanzees and macaques, by contrast, tend not to be willing to exert themselves so selflessly. Typically, even the young have to demand food or comfort. Interestingly, male marmosets were much more likely than females to display this largesse.

Aggression brings us to yet another hypothesis concerning the human disposition to cooperate, proposed by evolutionary theorist Samuel Bowles.[72] If ancestral groups (about 25–100 people) engaged in lethal intergroup competition, where the group successful in battle takes the resources of the vanquished, resource leveling (sharing the spoils of victory, food sharing beyond the family, and respect between males of one another's bonds with females) would be needed to reward those willing to risk life and limb. Resource leveling, and respect for others men's wives, helps to ensure future loyalty and decreases within-group competition. So, reasons Bowles, if clan warfare is accompanied by practices of resource leveling, the genes for altruism will spread through a population. The plausibility of Bowles's hypothesis depends on, among many other things, whether ancestral groups of hominins did engage in lethal intergroup competition, and certainly hard evidence is difficult to come by. On this question, his recent analysis of archaeological data suggests that around 50,000 years ago, violence did account for a remarkable number of deaths.[73] While at some sites there is no evidence of violent death, at others, about 46% died violently. Averaged across sites, about 14% appear to have died violently, a very high figure. Whether this is evidence of intergroup warfare is not settled. A further question for Bowles is whether a different explanation for altruism in women is needed, given that the selection pressure seems to be confined to men.

Bowles argues that ethnographic and historical data on hunter-gatherer societies living in conditions similar to those that probably obtained during the early appearance of humans also support the probability of significant warfare. The ecological conditions may be crucial to whether warfare was common or occasional. Warfare between Inuit groups is believed to have been virtually nonexistent before contact with Europeans, though the data indicate that warfare along the coast of Hudson Bay and James Bay between Inuit and Cree, who were culturally and linguistically very different, was not uncommon. Although separating fact from fantasy in early reports of Inuit life remains difficult, we do know that life was exceedingly harsh and precarious, and groups were small, varying between about 8 and 25 individuals. Inuit would kill a stranger, even another Inuit, caught within their territory, and would kill for revenge, but they appeared to engage in all-out wars between Inuit groups fairly rarely.[74] There was intermarriage between groups, so the presence of kin in other groups may also have deterred tribal conflict. The demands of the ecology and the constant battle against starvation may have meant that war was excessively costly, and save for the raids on the Cree for wives, it may have been counterproductive.

These four hypotheses regarding the evolution of human cooperation—loose hierarchy and relatively easygoing temperament, cooperative parenting expanding to cooperation with the group, sexual selection, and lethal intergroup competition—are not mutually exclusive, and given the paucity of evidence of human social life 300,000 years ago, it will be interesting to watch the fate of each as new data emerge.

• • •

In humans, the nature of social life changed enormously as the species began to exploit the benefits of agriculture over a strictly hunter-gatherer life. Agriculture and herding supports many more individuals, and groups can become larger without depleting the resources of the immediate areas. Trade can be conducted on a broader scale. New divisions of labor—goatherds, boatbuilders, carpenters—appear. And new social problems emerge; cultural practices, along with technology, become more complex. New ways of doing things emerge, including cooperation across clan boundaries. The conditions necessary for sociality depend on the brain's homeostatic emotions and the expansion within one's homeostatic ambit of offspring, kin, and affiliates. Sociality also depends on the brain's capacity to learn—by imitation, by trial and error, by conditioning, and by instruction. So far, little has been said about the contribution of genes to the brain organization that supports sociality. Chapter 5 will focus on genetic questions, and on what is, and is not, known about how genes influence our social behavior.

5. Networking: Genes, Brains, and Behavior

As a species of mammal, humans seem capable of impressive cooperation, especially among kin, but also among strangers, and especially when conditions permit and advantages are discerned. Regarding this capacity as "in our nature" has motivated a long list of evolutionary biologists and psychologists to speculate on the genetic basis for cooperation. One caution already on the table: quite a lot of human cooperative behavior may be explained by capacities other than cooperation biologically defined (i.e., as selected for). For example, strong sociable dispositions, along with the motivation to belong and learn social practices, may suffice to explain many cases of joint efforts.

What other factors might figure in the getting along and helping out? A capacity to defer gratification and suppress costly impulses (known as *executive functions*) is important in acquiring social skills and making cooperative behavior advantageous. Many humans are skilled in evaluating what is in their long- and short-term interests, and they frequently distinguish between genuine cooperation that might bring general benefits, and phony cooperation that is really exploitation by an ambitious profiteer. In addition, humans are well able to draw on past experience to find analogies to a current problem, and to then apply an analogous solution. These abilities are presumably among those Aristotle had in mind when, in his *Nicomachean Ethics*, he discussed in great detail the acquisition of social virtue and wisdom through experience.[1] Some of these capacities, jointly and severally, may go a long way in explaining many examples of human coopera-tion; for example, building a bridge to reach good pasture, which re-quires cooperation in moving logs and hoisting them into place. These considerations raise the possibility that cooperativity *as such* may not be causally linked to large effects by specific genes, even though the background neurobiological functions such as caring for offspring and mates, and the desire to avoid punishment and disapproval, are highly heritable. This would be rather like the discovery that while aggres-sion in fruit flies can be selected for in the lab, and hence is heritable, aggression *as such* is not linked to large effects by specific genes dedi-cated to the aggressive behavior. (More on this below.)

I am suggesting that caring—for self, kin and affiliates, for example—can frequently give rise to mammalian and avian behavior commonly called cooperative, and that the genetic background that contributes to caring circuitry may carry more of the explanatory bur-den for common instances of cooperation than previously supposed. On this analysis, cooperation, like aggression in defense of offspring, is a manifestation of attachment and caring. This does not rule out a specific genetic basis for cooperation. It does, however, invite circum-spection about *genes for cooperativity*, made more emphatic by recent attempts to link genes and behavior in the fruit fly, to which I shall now turn.

In their comprehensive and readable book *How Genes Influence Behavior* (2010), geneticists Jonathan Flint, Ralph Greenspan, and Kenneth Kendler list the criteria to be satisfied by a claim that "X is a gene for Y":

We can summarize as follows: if gene X has a strong, specific association with a behavioral trait or psychiatric disease in all known environments and the physiological pathway from X to Y is short or well-understood, then it may be appropriate to speak of X as a gene for Y. . . . Do genes have a *specific* effect on behavior? Almost certainly not.[2]

Genetic Networks

The relations between genes and behavior, as geneticist Ralph Greenspan observes,[3] are not one-to-one, not even one-to-many; they are *many-to-many*. The significance of this point, now broadly appreciated by geneticists, has been steadily eroding the idea of a big-effect gene for this or that specific behavior such as aggression or cooperation. Let's start with evidence for one-to-many mappings. *Pleiotropy*—when a gene plays a role in many different, and functionally distinct, aspects of the phenotype (traits the organism has)—turns out to be not the exception, but the *rule*.[4] Moreover, when a gene plays a role *both* in vital operations of the organism's body *and* in behavior, via brain circuitry, then it is subject to stringent selection constraints. That is, behavioral mutants still have to be viable and relatively normal.[5] If a mutation happens to produce a behavioral advantage, it must not mess up other bodily functions so much as to imperil viability. So if I am born a genius but the mutation enabling my genius results in a dysfunctional liver, my genius will go for nought. Only very rarely does a gene mutation yield results that are sufficiently positive that the organism's body and brain are advantaged in the struggle for life and reproduction.

The evidence indicates that most gene products (usually proteins but some can be RNA—ribonucleic acid) *do* play multiple roles, in body and brain. That is, the protein that a gene codes for may play a role in such diverse functions as building a liver, maintaining the inner membrane of the esophagus, sweeping up extra neurotransmitter at a synaptic site, and modification of a neuron's membrane during learning. Serotonin, for example, figures in cardiovascular regulation, respiration, circadian rhythm, sleep-wake cycles, appetite, aggression, sexual behavior, sensorimotor reactivity, pain sensitivity, and reward learning.[6] Depression has been associated with a short allele (variant of the gene) for the serotonin transporter protein, and the data are sometimes interpreted as meaning that having the gene causes depression. In fact, the effects are actually small, though statistically significant, and the presence of the short allele accounts only for 3–4% of the variation in the general population of the measures of depression, and 7–9% of inherited variance of the trait. This means that many other factors play an important role in the occurrence of depression.[7] This is not surprising. Consider that the physical trait of height in humans is associated with 54 known alleles, but collectively, they account only for 5% of the heritability of height. The rest is a mystery.

Here is a telling example of pleiotropy. In the early days of fruit fly genetics, it was widely believed that a single mutation to a gene called "dunce" affected just one capacity, namely associative conditioning (i.e., learning that one event predicts occurrence of another event; my dog Duff learned that jangling car keys in the morning predicts a walk to the beach). The *dunce* gene, it seemed, was the gene for associative conditioning, and was probably selected for the advantages accruing to those flies who could learn to associate one event with another. In the beginning at least, it really looked that way. Follow-up studies, however, show that the gene product (cyclic AMP phosphodiesterase) also plays a role in embryonic patterning, and in female fertility. This was surprising—female fertility and the capacity to learn a conditioned response would seem to have little to do with one another. They do not even seem to form a functional cluster, at least at the macro level. But genes are not one-trick ponies.

Given evolution's *modus operandi*—tinkering-opportunistically rather than redesigning-from-scratch—we should not expect our conception of functional categories at the macro level to map neatly onto genes and gene products.[8] Thus "capacity for conditioning" does not one-to-one-map onto *dunce*. In the very earliest stages of life on the planet, all the functions of a gene product such as cyclic AMP phosphodiesterase might have been more closely related, but as time and evolution moved on, structural branch points became increasingly elaborate and widely separated. Thus serotonin, perhaps handling only a single job in very simple organisms, gets recruited for new tasks, and ultimately ends up doing many things whose connections with each other are lost in our evolutionary past. Consequently the functions of the gene product can end up in very different categories. The various functions associated with the products of *dunce* may have something in common in the deep history of evolution, but that commonality cannot possibly be read off our conventional categorization of functions such as female fertility or associative conditioning. By and large, the strategy of trying to link a single gene to a particular phenotype has been superseded by the understanding that genes often form networks, and that a given gene is likely to figure in many jobs.

Now for the many-to-one-mapping problem, and the parable of fruit fly aggression. In fruit flies and mice, a connection between serotonin and aggression has been observed. Experimentally elevating levels of serotonin using drugs or genetic techniques increases aggression in the fruit fly; genetically silencing serotonin circuits decreases aggression. On the other hand, elevating levels of neuropeptide-F decreases aggression, and genetically silencing neuropeptide-F increases aggression.[9] These results are, moreover, consistent with experiments on the mouse, suggesting conservation of mechanisms for aggression through evolutionary change. One might even be tempted to think of the gene that expresses serotonin as the "aggression gene." Not so.

Over some twenty-one generations, Herman Dierick and Ralph Greenspan[10] selectively bred aggressive fruit flies (the little pugilists keep on fighting rather than quitting, and are thirty times more aggressive than the wild type). Since the flies had been bred for aggressive behavior, it was possible then to ask: What are the genetic differences between the aggressive and the docile flies? To do this, they compared the gene-expression profiles of the aggressive flies with those of their more docile cousins using molecular techniques (microarray analysis). (A gene is expressed either when it makes the protein it codes for, or, in the case of noncoding genes, it makes RNA. So for a coding gene, an increase in its expression means that more of the protein it codes for is produced. Gene expression may be regulated by yet other genes and their products, which may turn a gene off or on. Altering genes expression can alter the observable traits of an organism.)

If the gene for serotonin really was the key to levels of aggression in an organism, one would predict that the aggressive flies would have an increase in serotonin. The surprising result was that this is not what was observed in the analysis of gene expression. In fact, no single gene could be fingered as specifically associated with aggression. Gene expression differences between aggressive and wild-type fruit flies were found in about 80 different genes; the differences in expression in those identified were all quite small. Moreover, many of the 80 genes whose expression changed (up or down) are genes known to play a role in a hodgepodge of phenotypic events—cuticle formation, muscle contraction, energy metabolism, RNA binding, DNA binding, development of a range of structures including cytoskeleton. No single gene on its own seemed to make much difference, but collectively the changes in the 80 genes did somehow produce highly aggressive fruit flies. Not all of the 80 different genes are necessarily related to the aggressive phenotypes, since some are undoubtedly "hitchhiking" along with those that were selected.

The crux of "The Parable of Aggression in the Fruit Fly" can be summarized thus: there is no single, big-effect gene for aggression in the fruit fly. Of those many genes differentially expressed between the wild-type and aggressive lines, none were the genes involved in serotonin or neuropeptide-F expression. None were even other proteins in the serotonin-metabolism chain.[11] How can that be, given the earlier experiments showing that elevating serotonin levels enhances aggression? It seems puzzling, at least until one recalls the complexity of genotype-phenotype relationships Ralph Greenspan has emphasized; genes are part of networks, influencing and interacting with each other and with features of the environment.[12] One factor contributing to this complexity is that serotonin is a very ancient molecule, important, as noted above, in a motley assortment of brain and body functions, including sleep, mood, gut motility (such stomach and intestinal contractions), bladder functions, cardiovascular function, stress responses, induction of smooth muscle proliferation in lung vessel during embryological development, and regulating acute and chronic responses to low levels of oxygen (hypoxia).[13] The unsuitability of the label "aggression gene" is glaringly obvious. The diversity in serotonin's jobs helps explain how it is that changing its levels can have widespread effects all over the brain and body. For these changes can cascade into other effects, which may in turn exert an influence on aggressive behavior. The idea is not merely that things are complex, which they surely are, but that a gene product can have many roles, and genes interact in ways that are typical of a nonlinear dynamical system—more like the behavior of a flock of crows than that of clock. As Greenspan has remarked, "The wider the network of contacts a gene product makes, the more chances there are for an alteration in another gene to influence it."[14]

The complexities pile on. Because genes and their products are involved in the construction of body and brain, and because the nervous system interacts with the environment in a manner that in turn can cause changes in gene expression, it is improbable in the extreme that a situationally sensitive behavior such as aggression or cooperation can be causally linked to the presence of a single gene or even a couple of genes.[15]

As the developing organism interacts with the environment, gene expression may be upregulated or downregulated (more protein is made or less protein is made). Neuroscientist Eric Kandel was interested in whether there would be changes in gene expression when mice learned something, in this case, to associate a location with a mild foot shock, and found that there was. In comparing the brains of the conditioned mice with naïve mice, he found two genes that were highly expressed in the system mediating fear—in the lateral nucleus of the amygdala (needed for processing fear responses) and in the pathways carrying the fearful auditory signal to the lateral nucleus amygdala.[16] For another example, in young songbirds, gene expression of the gene *zenk* is triggered when the bird hears the song of its species, the gene product playing a role in the bird's learning the song of its own species.

Despair is not the lesson of this bewildering complexity. Nor is the lesson that genes do not affect behavior. They do, of course, and heritability studies in populations confirm that some traits are highly heritable. Height, for example, is strongly heritable, as are temperamental profiles (e.g., introversion, extroversion, and probably degrees of sociability), and the susceptibility to schizophrenia or alcoholism. The point is that *if* a certain form of cooperation, such as making alarm calls when a predator appears, has a genetic basis, it is likely to be related to the expression of *many* genes, and their expression may be linked to events in the environment.

Almost certainly social behavior in mammals depends on genes for oxytocin (OXT), oxytocin receptors (OXTR),[17] vasopressin (AVP), endogenous opiates, dopamine, and dopamine receptors, serotonin and serotonin receptors, as well as genes involved in the development of circuitry such as that supporting the extensive pathways of the vagus nerve through the body. *For starters*.

As Frances Champagne and Michael Meaney have shown, licking and grooming by the mother rodent has effects on the subsequent social behavior of the babies; pups who get plenty of licking and grooming are more socially adept than pups who do not.[18] Genes are part of a flexible, interactive network that includes other genes, the body, the brain, and the environment. But to quote Greenspan again, "Synergism and network flexibility make it easier to conceive of how new properties in behavior can emerge: tune up an allele here, tune down another one there, combine them with some other preexisting variants, and boom! You have a new behavior."[19]

Innate Moral Principles and Innate Moral Foundations

In humans, ecological conditions, accidents of history, and cultural practices result in striking diversity in social organizations, including that aspect we refer to as morality. Even so, at a general level of description, there are obvious common themes among social organizations regarding values. One the face of it, these appear to reflect similar general strategies for solving rather similar problems of living together. Courage in defense, cunning in the hunt, honesty in transactions, tolerance of idiosyncrasies, and willingness to reconcile—these are values touted in the stories not only of aboriginal tribes, but of agricultural and post-industrial people as well. Many groups share similar stories of vices: aggression gone sour, lust overwhelming good judgment, self-indulgence bringing ruin, ambition wreaking havoc, and miserliness leading to loneliness.

The generality of these themes does not entail that humans have a "hard-wired module" specifying particular kinds of social behavior, where the wiring-up is controlled by genes dedicated to producing that behavior. Although such a hypothesis cannot be absolutely ruled out, the complexity of gene-behavior relationships illustrated by "The Parable of Aggression in the Fruit Fly" suggests that aggression in the human, not to mention cooperation in the human, is unlikely to be associated with a few large-effect genes. Granting individual human differences, similarly organized brains facing similar problems are likely to land on similar solutions. Wood works well in boatbuilding, merriment eases social tensions, competitive games are less costly than fights. Languages may have emerged from similar pushes and pulls, without the help of a dedicated, new "language gene."[20]

Complexity in genes-brain-behavior interactions notwithstanding, the idea that morality is basically innate remains irresistible. As with many ideas that bob up again and again despite withering criticism, enough is right about it to attract adherents. There is no doubt that genes have a huge effect on our nature, but the problem is to say something meaningful about that relationship. The more distant one is from the hands-on study of genes, the greater the temptation to wave vaguely in the direction of genes and innateness and selection, as the source of an explanation for aspects of human behavior.

Plato, among the first to "solve" the problem of where values come from by invoking innateness, argued that we are born knowing the basic principles of morality, though he had to admit that the process of birth must entail some forgetting and introduces some weakness in the face of temptation. Fortunately, he thought, the innate knowledge is gradually recollected through time and experience, and in old age, if lucky, we can be knowledgeable once more about the Good. Plato had no decent theory to explain how our previous selves came by the knowledge in the first place, only pushing the problem back further. This remains a totally unsolved Platonic problem.

Recently, Marc Hauser, a psychologist and animal behavior scientist, defended the innateness approach to morality. Hauser thinks there are universals in human moral understanding—views about what is right and what is wrong—that obtain in all societies. These universals are, he contends, visible in the unreflective intuitions that people summon in addressing a specific moral issue. For example, Hauser finds that there is widespread agreement that incest is wrong, and that drinking apple juice from a brand-new bedpan is disgusting.[21]

Universals in moral intuitions, so Hauser's argument continues, are strong evidence of an innate physiological organization that, given normal brain development, typically yields those intuitions. Call these moral intuitions, *conscience*, or perhaps, with Hauser, products of the *moral organ*. Hauser's own view and research program are modeled on linguist Noam Chomsky's view on the origin of human language and language acquisition. Chomsky believes that the human brain is genetically equipped with a unique "language organ" specifying abstract principles of syntax that become more concrete with exposure to language. From this organ flows our grammatical intuitions, and our ability to learn specific languages. Hauser argues that humans likewise have a "moral organ" that specifies the universal principles of morality, and from which originates our moral intuitions about right and wrong: "we are born with abstract rules or principles, with nurture entering the picture to set the parameters and guide us toward acquisition of particular moral systems."[22] In emphasizing the hardwired aspect, Hauser says, "Once we have acquired our culture's specific moral norms—a process that is more like growing a limb than sitting in Sunday school and learning about virtues and vices—we judge whether actions are permissible, obligatory, or forbidden, without conscious reasoning and without explicit access to the underlying principles."[23]

We have already spent some time looking at genetic networks and gene-environmental interactions; we need to dwell a little more on the issue of exactly what is meant by "innate" in the context of behavior. An expression with a tortured history, "innate" is used to refer to a wide or a narrow range of phenomena, or much in between. A concertina concept—one that expands and contracts as the conversation and criticism fluctuate—*innateness* sometimes impedes clarity. To defend a hypothesis about innateness for a particular behavioral trait, what kind of factual evidence must be marshaled? As compactly stated by Flint, Greenspan, and Kendler early in this chapter,[24] one needs to identify the genes involved, show how they help organize neural circuitry, and then show the relation of the circuitry to the behavior. Lacking that— and invariably that is lacking in human studies—social scientists resort to identifying what is *innate* via behavior. How does that work? Sometimes the specification rests on the idea that for anything we can easily acquire through learning, the genes provide the brain with an *innate capacity*—a structural "readiness." *Anything?* Even reading, riding a bicycle, and milking a cow—all of which are typically easily learned, but cannot have been selected for in the evolution of the human brain?[25] Because such generality seems to bleed the meaning out of the term, *anything* has to replaced with a more adequate filter.

On a more restricted use of *innate*, it refers to those behaviors that are both "genetically programmed" and universally displayed by all individual that carry the relevant genes (and easily learned). Generally, of course, which genes are implicated is not known, and "easily learned" has, as noted, its own problems, so the heavy lifting falls to *universality*. Because there are not only gene-environment interactions, but also interactions between the developing brain and the environment within the uterus, some researchers find this proposed modification for *innate* too imprecise and too burdened with historical mistakes to be useful.[26]

According to Hauser, "our moral faculty is equipped with a universal moral grammar, a toolkit for building specific moral systems." Echoing Chomsky's claim that there are unlearnable languages, Hauser states further, "*Our moral instincts are immune to the explicitly articulated commandments handed down by religions and governments.*"[27] Hauser's optimism with respect to innate moral intuitions is perhaps inspiring, but it is truly hard to square with history and anthropology. Consider the many examples of human sacrifices as part of religious rituals, the vulnerability to propaganda, the willingness to go to war on a tide of jingoism, the nontrivial variability in moral customs concerning the status of women, torture during the various Inquisitions and wars, and most remarkably, the mass murder of Jews, Tutsis, Ukrainians, Poles, Lithuanians, and Native Americans, to name but a few of the massacres. Sadly, many of these practices did follow the exhortations and encouragement by governments and religions. One cannot but conclude that our *moral behavior* seems more susceptible "to the explicitly articulated commandments handed down by religions and governments" than what, according to Hauser, can be expected from a properly functioning moral organ. The question of evidence for Hauser's hypothesis is pressing.

Apart from concern about the semantic unsteadiness in *innate*, I also have reservations about what *universality*, when actually observed, implies. I suspect that the existence of common themes and styles in human behavior is not a reliable sign of a genetic basis for a specific behavior.[28] Let me explain. A universally (or more likely, *widely*) displayed behavior *may* be innate, but it may also just be a common solution to a very common problem.[29] For contrasting examples, note that blinking in reaction to a puff of air directed at the eye is a reflex. It appears to be a direct outcome of known brainstem circuitry, and is minimally affected by the environment, and minimally affected by training. If one feels compelled to use the concept of "hard-wired" in human behavior, this case may be as good as it gets. By contrast, making boats out of wood is common in cultures that have access to wood and a desire to move about on water.[30] Apparently, boat-making with wood is universal, and probably was used by earlier hominins to get themselves to Indonesia. But is it *innate*? Do we have a genetic basis for making boats? Do we have an innate "boat-making organ"?[31]

Probably not. Wood is just a good solution to the problem of making a boat, because it floats, is available in lots of places, and is moderately easy to work with. Logs can be lashed together, a large tree can be hollowed out with stone axes, and so forth. Making boats of wood is a reasonable solution to a problem; that is all it is. Or, as the late Elizabeth Bates famously pointed out, in all cultures, people feed themselves with their hands—not because they have an innate hand-feeding module programmed by the hand-feeding gene, but because given our physical equipment, eating with hands is a good solution to a problem. We could, if determined, eat with our feet, or just lean over and put our faces in our food (and we sometimes do). But using hands is an obvious, rather efficient way of getting the job done, and that convenience, given our equipment, is all that is needed to explain the universality of hand-feeding. Now for an example from the domain of morality.

Truth-telling is widely considered a virtue. This is plausibly related to the fact that for reasons pertaining to survival, humans value accurate predictions, and hence value being able to rely on one another for information regarding food sources, predators, how to make a boat, and so forth. Because our life and well-being depend on it, reliability is preferred over unreliability. A social practice that approves truth-telling and disapproves deception does not imply the existence of a special gene or a special module; it can be explained in terms of routine human problem-solving, given human intelligence and the platform for sociability. Seeing the practice this way also is consistent with the fact that humans are quite willing to deceive when conditions clearly require it, such as when prudence requires deceiving an enemy of the community. Spies, after all, are supposed to deceive, as are undercover police in a sting operation. And "white lies" in the service of social graciousness are absolutely required, according to Miss Manners. Which is why truth-telling is a social practice, not a strict rule. The impropriety of telling the truth on certain occasions is learned along with the practice of generally telling the truth. (See chapter 6, where the role of rules is more thoroughly explored.)

What these examples imply is that for these cases at least, no innate brain modules are needed—no boatbuilding or hand-feeding or truth-telling genes need be postulated. The logical point is simple: universality is *consistent* with the existence of an innate module, but it does not *imply* the existence of an innate module. Compelling evidence in addition to universality is needed. For some traits, it may be that *if* it is innate, then it is universal. But it would be a fallacy to say, well, the trait *is* universal, therefore it must be innate.[32]

Importantly, traits may be innate without being universal, as is lactase persistence in a subset of humans. Methodologically, such diversity in traits among populations can be a boon. As philosophers of science Jonathan Kaplan and David Buller both point out, if comparisons between populations regarding differential appearance of a trait can be linked to relevant differences in the ecology, then they can be linked to an adaptation for the trait in special ecological conditions.[33] Comparison of populations with and without light skin helped nail down the hypothesis that light skin allows for greater penetration of ultraviolet light, enhancing synthesis of vitamin D. This penetration is useful in latitudes far from the equator where the winters are long (and where light skin is common), and a handicap in latitudes closer to the equator where sunburn would be a problem. At least 100 genes have been implicated in skin pigmentation, so how exactly light skin emerged in populations that migrated into Europe is not completely understood. Still, this serves as a reminder that a trait may have a genetic basis but not be universal.

Here is the more general caution: when it comes to behavior such as displays of cooperation, as opposed to the eye-blink reflex, appealing to innateness is often minimally informative. That is because what mediates the behavior is neural circuitry, and neural circuitry, as we have seen, is the outcome of gene-gene, gene-neuron-environment, neuron-neuron, and brain-environment interactions. Without a doubt, genes have a huge role to play in what we are, but exactly what the role is remains to be clarified.

Learning, of course, greatly adds to the complexity of the picture. Neuroscientist Charles Gross observes that in some humans who pay a lot of attention to cars there are regions of the temporal lobe that respond differently to different models of cars—to Cadillac Seville versus Audi 5000 versus Ford Taurus.[34] This can be demonstrated using brain imaging techniques. Is such a region an innate "car" module? Obviously, car model identification was not selected for in our evolutionary history, though such a capacity may be highly advantageous these days. The temporal lobe, as Gross says, seems to be a general-purpose analyzer of visual forms that are relevant to how the animal makes its living. The basic lesson then is that working backwards from the existence of a certain behavior to a brain region that supports that behavior to the innateness of a function is, especially in animals that are prodigious learners, a project fraught with evidential hazard.

As things stand, it is clear that postulating "genes for" truth-telling, for example, has little to recommend it.[35] If, as described earlier, the relation between aggressiveness and genes in the fruit fly is complicated, then it is not surprising that the relation between genes and moral values espoused by humans, with their massive prefrontal cortex, their immaturity at birth, and the staggering amount of learning they do, looks to be very complicated indeed. [36]

Hauser is surely to be applauded for favoring scientific approaches in trying to discover the moral intuitions of the general public regarding certain moral dilemmas, and he does draw on a very broad sampling of opinion, to be sure. Nevertheless, the apparent universalities that he finds in responses to questionnaires maybe be partly owed to the simplicity, and lack of context, for many of the dilemma-stories subjects are asked to respond to. And as Philip Zimbardo has shown in his decades of careful work, a person's written response to a questionnaire may bear only a slight resemblance to what he or she would do if actually placed in a real situation. [37]

Consider one example from Hauser. Virtually everyone who fills out his questionnaire responds with disgust to the idea of drinking fresh apple juice out of brand-new hospital bedpan. But what is the context for this? If I were to consider the idea as I sit now at my desk, well fed and well hydrated, I would not find it appealing, obviously because of the association with urine. Suppose, however, I am desperately dehydrated, stranded in the desert, and (miraculously) a camel appears with the bedpan full of fresh apple juice strapped to its hump. Would I find drinking it disgusting? Not in the slightest. How would contemporary subjects respond to the idea of using salt obtained by evaporating urine? My guess is that they would respond with disgust. Yet the Aztecs, hard put to find salt, used that as a method. [38] Were I an Aztec in that circumstance, I am betting I would tuck into the salt with gusto, not disgust, just as the Aztecs likely did. [39] As both Aristotle and Confucius realized, context matters a lot, which is why they both considered moral knowledge to be rooted in skills and dispositions, not a set of rules or, in Hauser's terms, a "moral grammar."

So the further caution is this: the existence of one's own powerful intuition about what is disgusting or wrong is not evidence that the intuition has an innate basis. It is *consistent* with that possibility, but it is also consistent with the possibility that the intuition reflects a social practice picked up during childhood, and ingrained via the reward system.[40]

Moreover, as Cambridge philosopher Simon Blackburn points out in contrast to Hauser, many moral dilemmas are addressed not automatically and instantly, but reflectively, with long, thoughtful deliberation.[41] Sometimes they remain unsettled for extended periods of time. Jurists, and those in government, as well as ordinary people, may struggle long and hard over the right way to handle moral problems involving inheritance laws, charging interest on loans, taxation, organ donation, eminent domain, "mainstreaming" mentally handicapped children in school, euthanasia for the terminally ill, immigration policy, war, removing children from parents, and capital punishment. On these topics, instant intuitions may give answers that backfire, and fair-minded disagreement can persist for decades. Hauser's claim that moral judgment does not involve conscious reasoning may apply in some situations such as seeing a child choking at dinner, but it clearly does not apply in multitudes of other situations, such as whether to go to war against a neighboring country.

Attuned to the realities besetting actual moral deliberation and negotiation, Blackburn challenges Hauser's analogy between moral intuitions and linguistic intuitions: "So to sum up they [moral intuitions] are apparently *not abundant, not instant, not inarticulate, not inflexible and not certain.* Any similarity to language processing is therefore on the face of it quite slight, and so, I fear, may be the prospects for diving down to find hidden principles constraining them."[42] Blackburn's summary captures well the profound disanalogies between linguistic intuitions and moral judgment. It would perhaps be appropriate to add that the originating germ of the analogy (the so-called "language organ" and grammatical universals) is itself the subject of more than a little skeptical debate.[43]

Jonathan Haidt and Moral Foundations

Jonathan Haidt, a psychologist,[44] argues that human morality is based on five fundamental intuitions, where each corresponds to an adaptation to an ecological condition, and each has its characteristic emotion. His theory includes a hypothesis to the effect that evolution favored humans who displayed these five virtues. The list he offers consists of name-pairs for the domains of intuitions, matched with the adaptive behavior.

1. *harm/care*—protect and care for young, vulnerable, or injured kin
2. *fairness/reciprocity*—reap benefits of dyadic cooperation with non-kin
3. *ingroup/loyalty*—reap benefits of group cooperation
4. *authority/respect*—negotiate hierarchy, defer selectively
5. *purity/sanctity*—avoid microbes and parasites[45]

Itemizing fundamental virtues has a venerable history in philosophy. Socrates, for example, starts with five (wisdom, courage, moderation, piety, and justice), but on reflection, demotes piety from the list, on grounds that it is not really a human virtue, but something that could be safely left to the Oracle at Delphi. The list in the Buddhist *Abhidharma* invites us to avoid the "three poisons" (hatred, craving, and delusion) and their assorted derivatives, while adhering to "Four Noble Truths" (loving-kindness, compassion, appreciative joy, and equanimity).[46] Mencius, a classical Chinese philosopher (4th c. BCE), listed four overarching virtues: benevolence, righteousness, propriety, and wisdom.

Aristotle's list distinguishes between intellectual virtues and those he calls *virtues of character* or *ethical virtues*. Aristotle emphasized that establishing appropriate habits in early life was essential for practical wisdom." As a useful bit of practical wisdom, he suggested that choosing the middle ground between extremes of behavior was a reliable, though not infallible, guide to leading a virtuous life—a rule of thumb known as the Golden Mean (not to be confused with the Golden Rule: "Do unto others as you would be done by"). The Golden Mean counsels us that the middle ground is generally good: one should be neither reckless nor timid, but appropriately courageous; neither tight-fisted nor openhanded, but appropriately generous; neither wholly indulgent nor utterly abstemious, but moderate; and so forth. How to be *appropriate* is not something that is settled by applying a rule, according to Aristotle; it requires practical wisdom, acquired through experience and reflection.

The Stoics emphasized the importance of prudence, wisdom, cour-age, and moderation, among other virtues. In the Middle Ages, others, including Aquinas and Ockham, also listed virtues, but in contrast to Socrates, "obeying God" was high on the list. Each of Aesop's fables ends with a summary statement of a bit of moral wisdom, which could be paired with a corresponding virtue, often that of prudence or mod-esty or kindness—"The moral of the story is. . . ."[47] In later periods, thrift and hard work were emphasized alongside the other virtues, as in Benjamin Franklin's list of thirteen virtues and, much more recently, in William Bennett's list of ten virtues.[48]

So Haidt is in respectable, if fairly crowded, company. Neverthe-less, Haidt wants to do more than just make a respectable list in the company of others. He wants also to claim an evolutionary basis for why some moral intuitions on his list (e.g., fairness) are actually fun-damental and innate, while others (e.g., truth-telling, or staying-calm-and-carrying-on) are secondary. Haidt's strategy has three parts: (1) identify the basic domains of intuition from what is known about the evolutionary conditions of early humans. (2) Show that these value-dispositions are common across diverse cultures. (3) Show that each value-disposition has its unique "characteristic emotion," thus support-ing the idea that it was selected for, and that it is fundamental, not secondary.[49]

Although the ambition of Haidt's project is laudable, the execu-tion is disappointingly insensitive to the height of the evidence bar. No factual support from molecular biology, neuroscience, or evolutionary biology is marshaled for his substantive claims about basic domains of intuitions. A danger in the project is that inferring what behavioral traits were selected for in human evolution cannot be solved by a vivid imagination about the ancestral condition plus selected evidence about cross-cultural similarity, evidence that could be explained in many different ways.[50]

The problem can be illustrated with Haidt's inclusion of a purity and sanctity domain as fundamental. His idea is that in the evolution of the human brain, religions would have served the well-being of individuals in the group who adhered to the religion, and hence the inclination would have been selected for in the biological evolution of the human brain. According to this view, beneficial intuitions about cleanliness and purity, originally connected to food, quite naturally attached themselves to local religious practices and objects. The foregoing sketches Haidt's account of what he believes is an innate inclination to religious adherence, and is meant to help explain the widespread occurrence of religions.

The problem is, theories abound to explain religions in terms of natural selection, and the lack of substantiating evidence makes them equally unappealing. To illustrate, one hypothesis meant to explain religious behavior, popular among anthropologists and psychologists, refers to *costly signaling*, which is a behavior displayed as a way of signaling cooperative intent and reliability. Examples of costly signaling would be sacrifices of goats and chickens, or the renunciation of comforts such as warm baths, or of pleasures such as dancing or sex. Simplified, the idea is that individuals who join a group and willingly accept the group's renunciations (costly signaling) are identifiable as reliable cooperators. Benefits flow from group membership; costly signaling is the price we pay to be members, and it helps to deter cheaters and freeloaders, who, *ex hypothesi*, would not want to pay. According to the costly signaling hypothesis, willingness to display costly signals would be selected for in the evolution of the species, since individuals could use them to find one another, and to expand groups with strongly cooperative members. Thus religion—usually involving costly signals such as sacrifices and renunciations—emerges as an innate module.[51] This sounds like a reasonable account, except that the evidence for the "costly signaling" hypothesis is in embarrassingly short supply. As philosophers have shown, none of the versions of this view are both logically coherent and sufficiently well supported to appear solid.[52]

Other strategies for explaining the ubiquity of religions proceed by arguing that in-group bonding occurs during religious rituals, enhancing attachment and loyalty, and that religion is thus a by-product of social bonding. Consequently, religious dispositions were selected for owing to the benefits of strong in-group bonds. This was advantageous in various aspects of social life where cooperation was needed. A somewhat different theory is that there are close links between religions and war. The motivating observation is that gods and spirits of war are very common, along with rituals with connections to war and fighting, and rewards for courageous fighters. Success in war, in both attack and defense, is a selective advantage, and religion aids a war effort.[53] Others have claimed that because people who had religious dispositions were on the whole healthier, the disposition to religion was selected for.[54] Though their arguments have been challenged and though there are some data showing that patients engaged in a religious "struggle" may actually be less healthy,[55] this link to health remains attractive to many people as a justification for religious faith.[56]

Another popular cluster of hypotheses claims that the disposition to religious beliefs is not selected for as such, but as a by-product of various other functions, such as attachment to parents, the wish for help in distress, and the inclination to explain mysteries and catastrophes by expanding one's attribution of mental states from the domain of observable humans to a domain of unobservable Others. Since religions are stunningly various, and deities come in all shapes, powers, and numbers (including zero), no single explanation along these lines holds much promise of doing the trick. Rather, a skein of interlocking explanations for different aspects of behavior that gets called "religious" may be more serviceable, in something like the way that many different things can be called music.[57] In any case, the plethora of selection theories to explain the prevalence of religious beliefs, none adequately supported by evidence so far, shows why leery evolutionary biologists and geneticists have shelved umpteen theories about innate modules as "just so" stories.[58] Speculations are of course useful in inspiring experiments, and are not to be discouraged. The point is, I prefer not buy into one, or be asked to, until some results bear upon its truth.

The classical problem that bedevils all innateness theories of behavior is that in the absence of supporting evidence concerning genes and their relation to brain circuitry involved, the theories totter over when pushed. Haidt, for example, relies quite heavily on whether or not a skill is easily learned to demarcate skills the brain is innately "prepared for" and those that it is not so prepared for.[59] But how do you defend, without resorting to ad hoc fixes, the innateness of some "easily learned" things while excluding other "easily learned" things, like riding a bicycle, tying a reef knot, putting on shoes, or fishing for trout with a worm on a hook? Conversely, learning skills of self-control, arguably something the brain probably is "prepared for," is often *not* easy. Ease of learning of a skill is *consistent* with innateness, but it does not *imply* it. The problems facing claims about the innateness of foundational moral behaviors are daunting, and without strong evidential support, the innateness claims are left dangling.

• • •

Aristotle, in his discussions of morality, emphasizes social skills as yielding the flexibility, aptness, and practicality required for flourishing in the social domain. In his view, the exercise of social skills depends on acquiring the appropriate habits, and can be greatly influenced by the role models, social practices, and institutions one encounters in daily life. An essential component of normal sociality involves our ability to attribute mental states to others. Without that capacity, we cannot empathize with their plight, nor understand their intentions, feelings, beliefs, and what they are up to. By and large humans are adepts in empathizing, and more generally, in "reading minds"—knowing what others feel, intend, want, and so forth. When the capacity begins to fail, as in frontotemporal dementia, which involves the degeneration of neural tissue in the frontal and temporal cortices, the effect is truly catastrophic, reminding us of how deeply important are the skills that we generally exercise effortlessly, fluently, and routinely. In the next chapter, I shall look more closely at what is known about the neuro-biology of understanding minds—others' and one's own.

6. Skills for a Social Life

The social world and its awesome complexity has long been the focus of performances—informally in improvised skits around the campfire, and more formally, in elaborate productions by professionals on massive stages. Among the cast of characters in a play, there is inevitably a wide variation in social intelligence, sometimes with a tragic end, as in *King Lear*. Comedy too is often wrapped around the contrasts between the socially adept and the socially bunglesome. A painfully funny character, such as Basil Fawlty (played by John Cleese in *Fawlty Towers*), reminds us of the agony caused by a foolish lie that has to be protected with increasingly intricate subterfuge to ward off more serious troubles, or by the brief lapse in self-control when dealing with an annoying customer. Basil's cooler and socially skilled wife Sybil is the foil, and her hotelier's professionalism makes more vivid the wholly unnecessary social jams into which Basil regularly gets himself stuck. What adds to the humor is that poor Basil is rather endearing, whereas Sybil, whose sincerity is often in doubt, is not. What are the differences in the brain between the socially skilled and the socially clumsy? What are social skills? How did the human social game come to be so complex, so subtle and full of shades upon shades of meaning?

In the front of the brain resides the prefrontal cortex (PFC), a large stretch of cortex whose most anterior region is behind the forehead.[1] It is the PFC, and its pathways to emotional brain structures, that yields the intelligence in human social behavior. When, after a stupid mistake, we slap our foreheads, we are giving a bit of a rattle to the PFC.

In the evolution of the hominin brain, the PFC became greatly expanded, and is much larger relative to body size in humans than in our mammalian relatives such as monkeys (see figure 6.1). The human PFC differs not just in size, but also in the density of major pathways connecting it to sensory areas in the posterior parts of the cortex.[2]

Neuroscientists think that the selective advantages of the larger PFC included greater capacity to predict, both in the social and in the physical domain, along with a greater capacity to capitalize on those predictions by deferring gratification and exercising self-control.[3] This has enabled greater flexibility in response to what is going on in the world, releasing us from the stock responses to threat and pain seen in evolutionarily simpler mammals such as rodents. With greater predictive capacities come greater opportunities to manipulate, in both the social and physical domains.

The cortical structures crucial to movement and behavior are also in the frontal cortex, just behind the PFC, and complex cognitive-motor skills rely on coordination between the frontal lobe and subcortical structures such as the basal ganglia. Altogether, Mother Nature seems to have found a winner in the PFC, and owing to its role in so many higher functions, the human PFC has been called "the organ of civilization."[4] Unfortunately, the mechanisms whereby the neuronal circuits in the frontal cortex perform this array of functions are not yet well understood, though neuroscientists have unearthed some essential elements in the story. Anatomists have shown that the prefrontal structures are densely connected to evolutionarily older subcortical structures such as the amygdala, hypothalamus, basal ganglia, and

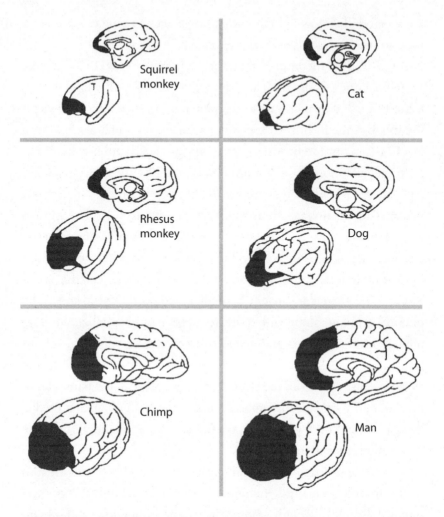

Figure 6.1. The dark area corresponds to the prefrontal cortex in each of the six species shown. Two views are shown: lateral-frontal (as though looking from the side and front), and medial, so the extent of the prefrontal cortex on the inner aspect of the hemisphere is represented. Not to scale. Reprinted from Joaquin Fuster, *The Prefrontal Cortex*, 4th ed. (Amsterdam: Academic Press/Elsevier, 2008). With permission from Elsevier.

nucleus accumbens, and are closely tied to emotions, feelings, sensation, drives, and the general state of the body.[5] A new anatomical technique, *tensor diffusion imaging* (TDI), is particularly advantageous in this study, since unlike traditional anatomical techniques, it can be used on living subjects, including humans.[6] TDI research reveals a pattern of connectivity common throughout the cortex, including the PFC: dense local connections, sparse distant connections, making for a "small world" configuration overall; not everything is connected to everything else, but via "well-connected" neighbors, a series of short hops allows you to reach everyone else.[7]

Careful clinical observations of stroke patients and patients with localized damage to the PFC have revealed correlations between damage to particular areas and particular deficits in function suffered by those patients. These studies have helped to map the functional organization of this large cortical territory. For example, damage to the orbitofrontal areas (roughly, the cortex above the orbits of the eyes) can result in hyperactivity, deficits in the evaluation of environmental cues, lack of empathy, reduced aggression in the face of threat, and emotional and social withdrawal. Prefrontal lobotomies, performed almost routinely on difficult patients until the mid-1950s, typically left subjects rather listless, with blunted emotional response.[8] Neuropharmacological research on the role of dopamine and norepinephrine and their receptors shows that PFC functions are highly sensitive to changes in levels of these neurotransmitters, changes that affect attention, mood, social behavior, and normal stress responses.[9] Serotonin is also a key player in the neurotransmitter story, especially in aspects of self-regulation and impulsive choice.[10] Neuroscientists have also shown that decreases in serotonin correlate with increased rejection of unfair offers in a game transaction, a finding that begins to probe the subtlety of the PFC.[11] During maturation the PFC lags behind all other cortical areas, and in humans some stages of PFC neural development are not mature until adulthood, a finding that seems consistent with the ordinary appreciation that in their social behavior and their capacity for self-control, adolescents are not yet fully mature.

It would be wonderful if this chapter could explain the neural substrate for complex social behavior, elucidating mechanisms involved in the behavior at the level of both macro- and micro-circuitry. Unfortunately, neurobiological knowledge has not caught up to our wishes.

In all aspects of neuroscience, prodigious gaps in our knowledge still stare out at us, and the PFC is especially difficult territory to study. The PFC is high up in the brain's processing hierarchy, and gets highly processed input from all over the brain.[12] Activity in an individual PFC neuron can be hard to interpret—does the activity relate to an emotion, to attention, to a sensory stimulus, to something held in working memory, to something expected in the future, to preparation for a movement? Or, quite possibly, to some combination of those factors? If an experimenter can control the known input to a neuron, as is possible for neurons in the visual cortex, meaningful results about the role of the neuron are more likely to be teased out. By controlling and monitoring input to a neuron in the visual cortex, neuroscientists have found neurons that, for example, are reliably responsive when and only when the stimulus is a bar of light moving up, others are highly responsive when and only when the bar of light is moving down, and so forth for all compass points. Building on this strategy, neuroscientists have been able to investigate neurons further up in the processing hierarchy, such as those that draw a conclusion about direction of motion as evidence accumulates about a visual stimulus.[13]

Studying the motor cortex has the inverse problem: although it is challenging to know exactly what the inputs to a neuron mean, if its output can be reliably correlated to specific behavioral responses, such as the movement of the thumb, then the experimenter can use that information to sort out the neuron's job. In the PFC, the main finding so far, using techniques for recording the activity of individual neurons, involves the dorsolateral PFC (put your hand between your ear and your temple; inside is the dorsolateral PFC).[14] This was done in the rhesus monkey. Some neurons in this area have been shown to hold information during a working memory task. If the task is to remember the location of a light on a grid after the light goes off, neurons in the dorsolateral PFC become active, and are spatially selective. Some will be active if the light was in the upper right, others if it was in the lower left, and so forth. Their activity drops once the monkey is allowed to point on the screen to where the light had been. But what about the role of the PFC in aspects of social behavior? What is the neural basis for compassion or for self-control or social problem-solving?

A variety of techniques have been used to good effect in investigating how the PFC works, but in studying human PFC function, the most common technique is *functional magnetic resonance imaging* (fMRI), greatly valued because it is noninvasive: no implantation of electrodes, no lesions, no cooling or radioactivity. Briefly, here is how it works. Magnetic resonance imagining gives a static picture of a person's insides, based on changes at the subatomic level that happen when the person enters the very strong magnetic field. The *functional* MRI technique builds on this by exploiting a lucky magnetic property of the blood: there is a difference in the magnetic properties of blood carrying oxygen versus blood whose oxygen has been taken up by cells (deoxygenated blood). This difference, called *blood-oxygen-level-dependent* (BOLD) contrast, can be picked up by detectors. The signals are averaged over time (a few seconds).

These changes would not be terribly interesting save for the fact that the BOLD signal correlates with the average level of activity of cells in a volume of neural tissue, perhaps less than a cubic millimeter in size, depending on the strength of the magnet used. The more active the neurons are, the more oxygen they use, and the BOLD signal reflects this, hence giving an indirect measure of physiological properties. Although neural activity is not measured directly by the BOLD contrast, on the assumption that the indirect measure is a good reflection of average neural activity in a small volume (a *voxel*: like a pixel, only, a small *cubic* volume), a researcher can use this fact to design experiments to investigate brain activity during a specific task, such as looking at a smiling happy face versus looking at a frowning face. To show the location of regions explored in the experiments, colored patches corresponding to the strength of the BOLD signal are superimposed on an anatomical image of the subject's brain. A great deal of care must go into both the design of the experiment and the analysis of the data collected in order to get meaningful results, but especially in the last few years, experiments using fMRI have been improving markedly.

Although fMRI is a tremendously powerful technique for studying brains of healthy humans, to understand results using the technique it is important to be aware of its limitations, which are occasionally obscured in reports of an fMRI experiment by the popular media. Typically the actual changes in the BOLD signal detected in fMRI experiments are very small, and the use of color, added to aid the visibility of the data, can mask this fact. If the picture of the brain shows one region colored red and another green, a casual reader might assume that the changes are pretty big, though in fact they may be tiny. In one coloring convention used by researchers, only the region where changes are seen is given any color, leaving the rest of the brain black. This is convenient for those in the field, but it has led students to believe that in the experimental condition, only the region in color was active, while the rest of the brain was snoozing. That inference is quite wrong, and the colored region merely represents change from a baseline of activity in that single region. Lots of activity was undoubtedly going on elsewhere, much of which likely supports the neuronal business in the region that is colored, but unless the activity level *changed*, it would not be represented in the picture.

An fMRI scanner with a spatial resolution of one cubic millimeter is a scientific thrill, relative to techniques available twenty years ago. Nevertheless, it is sobering to realize that in a cubic millimeter of cortical tissue, there are approximately 100,000 neurons and roughly a billion synapses.[15] The BOLD signal cannot of course monitor the changes in the activity of individual neurons—some up, some down, some unchanged—within a given cubic millimeter. At most, it reflects the aggregate activity over a few seconds. Nor can it address what operations (computational steps) are being carried out by the networks of neurons in a given voxel.

Moreover, some of the neurons in a cubic millimeter will have only short local connections, while others will have connections that are many centimeters in length and hence go beyond the confines of the population represented in the voxel. Some will be receiving input from elsewhere, some will be sending it elsewhere, but the BOLD signal is not sensitive to information flow. Observing an fMRI signal showing increased activity in a small area is a bit like hearing an increasingly loud hubbub in the rumpus room, but not knowing what each of the twenty children is up to. Moreover, even though there is no discernible hubbub in the kitchen, absence of hubbub does not mean absence of mischief. In short, fMRI does not reveal what is going on at the micro level of neurons and their networks. Without that, getting to the bottom of the operations and business of the PFC is problematic. Nevertheless, to repeat, fMRI is a wonderfully important technique for studying brain organization in humans, allowing us to see, for example, where there are differences between the brains of psychopaths and the brains of control subjects.[16]

One effect of converting the analysis of fMRI data to easily visualizable form is that pictures of brains with colored patches corresponding to a subject's executing specific tasks such as recognizing a car model (Cadillac Seville or Ford Crown Victoria) foster the idea that the cortex has relatively autonomous modules or centers, such as a module that is dedicated to recognizing distinct car models. Although the brain does display regional specialization, the idea of an autonomous module is substantially stronger than a specialized region, as it implies that the neurons in a module are dedicated to just that task and that the task is accomplished just by those neurons. The hypothesis that the cortex is made up of autonomous modules inspired some psychologists to claim that the brain is organized like a Swiss army knife, where each tool is autonomous relative to the others.[17] A major anatomical reason against this is the looping nature of the pathways—forward and back and sideways, long and short. Everywhere in the cortex we see convergence and divergence of information.[18] The autonomous module story may be consistent with existing fMRI data, but it does not get strong support from it. The region picked out is after all just one that consistently differs between the resting state and the task state (e.g. identify the car model). Unless that region got input from many other brain areas, the function (identifying the car model) under study could not be accomplished. In the brain, connectivity is crucial, and looping pathways, the rule. All of which dims the prospects for modularity in a strong "Swiss army knife" sense.[19]

Devising revealing techniques is not the only problem facing researchers of the PFC. In a deep sense, we are not sure *what* the jobs of the PFC really are: do we have the right vocabulary? Interpreting lesion and fMRI data typically entails deploying the familiar theory-of-mind categories, such as deferring gratification and self-control, yet we must question whether those categories are appropriate to capture what is going on from the point of view of the brain. For the early stages of visual cortex, by contrast, categorical probity is less of a problem. One can reasonably say, for example, that a neuron is tuned to respond to vertical direction of motion of a stimulus. It is less obvious, however, that expressions such as "deferring gratification" or "jumping to a conclusion" or "irrational fear" are really honored by brain circuitry. Do terms such as *weakness of will* or *strength of will*, for example, actually correspond to functionality in the PFC?

For botanists, the term *weed* does not really capture a category honored in the world of plants; its application depends greatly on human interests that may vary idiosyncratically and according to completely extraneous criteria. Some people call dill a weed, others cultivate it as an herb. Similarly, in the context of mind and brain, some terms, such as *decision-making* or *response inhibition*, likely do map onto brain circuitry, but other terms drawn from our behavior-level vocabulary, while useful in the day-to-day business of social life, may map poorly, if at all, onto the circuitry of the PFC. This theoretical worry becomes a concrete worry for neuroscientists who study the PFC, and who are trying to sort out the terms that do have explanatory traction from others that may be unable to get a precise neural grip, like *nervous breakdown*, which likely involves a semi-overlapping range of rather different causes, or *strength of will*, which likewise may not correspond to a single brain property.[20]

In the spirit of pragmatism and prudence, we will take a hard look at certain fashionable ideas about links between social understanding and neuronal mechanisms, especially those concerning the neural basis for attributing mental states to self and others (*theory of mind*) and concerning *mirror neurons* (to be explained anon). Common convictions about how mirror neurons explain skills in mental attribution have taken off in a way that leaves the evidence in the dust, and hence it may be useful to subject this idea to tough tire-kicking to determine what is really solid. Before that, however, we'll set the stage by looking at central aspects of social cognition, including acquiring a conscience. Toward the end of the chapter, we will also consider whether a link has been established between autism and faulty mirror neurons. We'll look at a fascinating social behavior known as *unconscious mimicry*, and explore a possible explanation for why humans, and some other social birds and mammals, so regularly and continually devote a lot of energy to it.

Social Knowledge, Social Learning, Social Decision-Making

The social life of primates is much more complex than that of rodents. In baboon troops, for example, social status depends on the ranking of the *matriline*—the lineage that passes from mother to daughter—into which one is born. Baboon troops are matriarchal; young male baboons leave the natal troop, whereas the females stay at home. Each animal understands in what matriline every animal belongs, how the matrilines are ranked relative to each other, and who ranks where within each matriline (older children are higher than younger ones).[21] Grooming relationships, threats, and specific vocalizations depend greatly on one's position in social space. Keeping track of who is who in the troop, of everyone's reputation, and of what sorts of expectations others have of oneself and of assorted others, involves a lot of social knowledge. The greater the capacity to make good social predictions and decisions—other things being equal—the greater the chances of well-being; in turn, the greater the chances of successful reproduction.

The social life of humans, whether in hunter-gatherer villages, farming towns, or cities, seems to be even more complex than that of baboons or chimpanzees. Typically humans have detailed knowledge of the character, temperament, kin relationships, and reputations of a lot of individuals.[22] In addition, humans are particularly skilled in adjusting behavior depending on context—at weddings, funerals, trade fairs, in a catastrophic situation, in the hunt, at work, at war, and so on. Knowledge about how to behave in diverse contexts is often picked up without explicit instructions of the relevant conventions. Although the motivation to acquire knowledge of social practices may emerge from the brain's dispositions to want to belong and to dislike separation, specific facts and skills are acquired. As with nonhuman animals, some people may be able to learn better or faster or more efficiently than others.

Human are consummate imitators, perhaps to a greater extent than any other mammals.[23] The capacity to imitate a skill learned by an elder puts the young human at a singular advantage: it does not have to learn everything by trial and error.[24] A child can learn from elders how to make fire and keep it going, how to stalk an elk, how to prepare for winter, how to set a broken bone. Jointly, the drive to learn by imitation and the inclination to upgrade that knowledge with new ideas is what yields the gradual accumulation of clever ways of doing things that can be passed on from one generation to the next. That is, it yields culture.

Humans, though impressive social learners, are not alone in learning from conspecifics. Parrots, cockatoos, mynah birds, finches, and sparrows are also adept imitators, and learn complex songs. Mockingbirds in our neighborhood sometimes give quail calls, then switch to finches, then make the sound of a telephone ringing. Some birds, such as the blue manakin of Argentina, learn complex dancing movements and compete for females through dance displays.[25] Bottlenose dolphins imitate the behaviors of their trainers,[26] and young predators such as cougars and bobcats do learn from their parents how to stalk and kill prey, and where to find them. The mother cougar will bring a maimed rabbit back to the den for the young to learn on. Veteran meerkats bring scorpions with the stinger removed to the home site so that the young can practice in safety. Andrew Whiten, Victoria Horner, and Frans de Waal, in carefully controlled experimental studies of chimpanzee "cultural transmission," also found that chimpanzees learned a novel foraging strategy by watching a skilled chimpanzee, while chimpanzees not able to observe the skill did not figure out the method.[27] (As they remark, it is essential in studying animal imitation that the behavior chosen for the animals to imitate is something that is ecologically relevant—something that the animals care about.) Field observations by anthropologists reveal that a particular group of baboons may have its own local customs, as when males hold one another's testicles (perhaps a trust ritual) when preparing for an aggressive raid on higher-ranking males. White-faced capuchin monkeys at the Lomas Barbudal Monkey Project in Costa Rica also have unique local traditions, such as fingering each others' eyeballs and sucking each others' fingers, or games where one monkey bites off a hank of fur of another monkey, and then the two engage in playful possession struggles.[28] Neonatal imitation has been observed in rhesus macaques,[29] and facial mimicry in young orangutans at play.[30]

For anecdotal evidence involving dogs, I offer this: I regularly walk our pair of golden retrievers on the golf course in the early morning before the first golfers appear. With significant effort, I trained the first pair to stay out of the sand traps and off the greens (there is a fairly fine distinction between greens and fairways, unless you are a golfer, but it pertains mainly to mowing level). When one died at 13, we got a second pair of pups. They quickly became attached to old Max, and he to them. When we began walks on the golf course, I expected to have to train Duff and Farley as I had the first pair. They did not need training from me, however, and simply did not go on the greens or into the traps. This behavior continued unchanged even after Max died a few months later. I never did see anything that I could definitely identify as imitative behavior, so if indeed they copied Max, it must have been somewhat subtle.

Learning Social Skills

Born with very immature brains, human juveniles are dependent on parents and willing others for an extended period. The benefit of immaturity at birth is that developing brains can exploit interactions with the environment to tune themselves up to the myriad ways of whatever physical and social world they find themselves in. Playing in those worlds, fooling around and goofing off, can lead to discoveries that are useful. Play in young predators is clearly associated with behavior they will later hone for killing prey, mating, and defending themselves.[31] From the perspective of evolution, learning has clear advantages in efficiency and flexibility over having it all "built in."[32]

In all highly social mammals, juveniles must learn to get along in the group, first with their mother and father, later with siblings, cousins, and so forth. The teething infant learns not to bite the mother's breast, the toddler learns to avoid the cantankerous uncle, children must learn to take turns, tolerate frustration, play fair, do their chores and so forth.

Acquiring a Conscience

As we grow up, we get approval for conforming to, and disapproval for transgressing against, social practices, and we feel pleasure or pain accordingly.[33] Early moral learning is organized around prototypes of behavior, and relies on the reward system to make us feel emotional pain in the face of some events (e.g., stealing), and emotional joy in the face of others (e.g., rescuing).[34] Through example, the child comes to recognize the prototype of fairness, rudeness, bullying, sharing, and helping. His understanding is also shaped by the clan's gossip, fables, and songs. As philosopher Simon Blackburn remarks,

> The emotional and moral environment in which children grow up is pervasive and many-faceted, carefully engineered by their caregivers, replete with soap operas, stories, sagas and gossip full of villains and heroes, retailed with smiles and frowns and abundant signs of esteem and dislike, and gradually entered by practise, imitation, correction, and refinement.[35]

Once a child has internalized local practices and knows what is expected, merely contemplating cheating or stealing is likely to be accompanied by images of consequences, and when those include social disapproval, the pain system will be active, if only in a low-level fashion. One might say that the child thus recognizes that the plan is wrong, or that his conscience tells him that doing the action would be wrong (figure 3.8, page 51, shows the reward system).

Because the generalized pain of shunning and disapproval is so aversive, and the pleasure of approval and belonging so rewarding, what is learned regarding social practices has a correspondingly strong emotional valence. So strong are these feelings about what is right and wrong that they may be regarded as having the status of divine origin, and the practices, as objective and universal. The practices of one's own clan can appear to be absolute and rational; differing practices can appear to be barbaric and irrational.

On the whole, the internalization of social standards via the reward/punishment system probably serves human social groups quite well. Individuals will risk quite a lot, sometimes even their lives, in defense of the group, or for a principle such as the abolition of slavery or even the idea of heaven. This internalization also means that prevailing practices may have substantial inertia, and can be changed only quite slowly, bit by bit. When the practices embody long-acquired wisdom, this can be beneficial. When conditions require a change, this inertia may be a detriment. Despite realizations that change would be beneficial, for example that the education of females enhances group economic prosperity, attitudes change slowly; but they can change, more typically in the young than in the old, more likely when there is wide exposure to non-kin values.[36]

Some ingrained attitudes, such as hostility to a particular out-group, in the form of racism, for example, can be particularly resistant to change. In these instances, deep internalization of social practices may not serve the group well, but instead contribute to wrenching instabilities, and many forms of cost, social and otherwise. In recent times, ethnic conflict in Rwanda and the Balkans has reminded us that out-group hostility can be disastrously entrenched.

Attributing Mental States to Self and Others

If we can learn to predict the behavior of others, we can often anticipate and avoid trouble or take advantage of foreseen opportunities. In predicting complex behavior, it is highly advantageous to interpret others' behavior as an expression of their inner mental states. Thus we might explain someone's error as a misperception or as a failure to pay attention; we might predict someone's participation in the upcoming defense of the village on the basis of his being highly motivated to protect his family.

Interpreting others' behavior in terms of their mental states such as intentions or perceptions can increase the effectiveness of predictions compared to the strategy of merely associating a particular bodily movement with a particular outcome (e.g., a hand raised gets associated with lights going out). Here is one reason why: the very same movement can be the outcome of very different intentions. For example, *thumbs up* can convey any number of things, depending on local conventions: some soccer players use it as an apology for an error; in kayaking, we use it to mean "let's go," as do pilots on aircraft carriers; the Romans used it to mean "let the gladiator live"; in Middle Eastern countries it can mean the equivalent of "up yours." Thus, predicting what you will do next is more effective if I have the capacity to interpret your behavior in terms of your inner intentions or feelings rather than just associating specific movements with particular outcomes. Ascending to this more abstract form of representation requires that background information about desires and beliefs, about reputation and context, and lots more besides, goes into the construction of the abstract representation of what the other person intends. From the opposite direction, the same intention may be executed by quite different means—I may drink by bending over a fountain, scooping water from a stream into my hands, raising a glass, or letting rain fall in my open mouth.[37] I may cheat in a thousand different ways, or cooperate in a thousand different ways. Once again, interpretation of what you are doing and going to do in terms of goals and intentions is more abstract and much more effective than merely associating specific movements with particular outcomes.

Not only is the accuracy of predictions increased, but having a systematic framework for attributing mental states opens up a whole new realm of understanding that in turn makes for yet more sophisticated interactions. Here is an artificially simple case to convey the flavor of what I mean: if I know that you can see the toddler walking toward the lake, and I know that you want to make sure she is safe if she goes swimming, and that you believe I will not act as lifeguard on this occasion, then I can predict you will walk with the toddler to the lake. If I know that you do not see the toddler walking toward the lake, I predict you will continue on your way to the garden, and I will need to alert you to do otherwise. The point is, by drawing on the systematic connections between various mental states, I have a powerful tool for navigating my social world and for reaching further into the social future. In view of these benefits, one might regard having a theory of mind—having the skills to attribute mental states to self and others—in terms of *representational practices* that support effective prediction and explanation.

Some people are more highly skilled than others in very complex social situations, such as department meetings or political conventions. For example, Jon Stewart (host of *The Daily Show*) is exceptionally skilled in sizing up the interplay of feelings, fears, expectations, and perceptions of his guests, in addition to having good background information, and thus he is able to smoothly guide conversation in insightful and often disarming ways. It is precisely the systematicity of the framework for attributing mental states that has encouraged application of the name "theory of mind," for the parts are knitted together into a dynamic whole as are the parts in a scientific theory.

Humans are skilled in attributing goals, desires, intentions, emotions, and beliefs to each other. We can envision the world from another's perspective, and we can imagine scenarios for the future. We also empathize with the plight and pains of others. Judging from the behavior of monkeys, chimpanzees, and scrub jays, humans are evidently not alone in achieving representational power in predicting what others are up to via a capacity for attributing mental states to others.[38]

The capacity to attribute mental states to others can be more or less rich, more or less sophisticated. Rhesus monkeys may be fairly accurate in attributing simple goals and feelings, but they are weaker than humans or chimpanzees in attributing complex goals. Dogs, who are bred to be sensitive to human purposes, can seem uncannily adept in predicting what an owner wants or will do. Moreover, though language may add to the sophistication of the representational schema, language is not necessary, at least for a rudimentary version of mental attribution—jays and chimpanzees lack language. Moreover, since children are able to learn the language of mental attribution, they likely have some representational skills already in place on which to build. Among psychologists, "mind reading" is sometimes the preferred name for the capacity, but because the expression seems to connote more in the way of cognitive accomplishment than the data warrant, I find it preferable to use a more modest expression, "the capacity for mental attribution."[39]

The questions I want to focus on now are these: What is known about the neural mechanisms that underlie the various skills involved in attributing mental states to others, and to oneself? Assuming that this capacity attributes many interlaced components (intentions, beliefs, feelings, desires, and so forth) that form something like a coherent representational schema, what are the internal dynamics of this schema? In what does its coherence consist?

Mirror Neurons and Mental Attribution (Theory of Mind)

In pondering the neural mechanisms for understanding others' mental states, many cognitive scientists have been greatly encouraged by the discovery of *mirror neurons* in the rhesus monkey.[40] The discovery was made at the University of Parma, in the lab of Giacomo Rizzolatti, and was first reported in 1992.[41] Mirror neurons are a subset of neurons in the frontal cortex of the monkey (specifically, a region called F5, in the premotor cortex and in the inferior parietal cortex (IP) (figure 6.2 shows the locations of these areas) that respond *both* when the monkey sees another individual grasp an object (e.g., I put food in my mouth), *and* when it performs that action itself (e.g., it puts food in its own mouth). A minority of F5 neurons tested, about 17%, showed this property. Meaningless actions, actions without an object, the mere presence of an object, or action by a hand where the rest of the body cannot be seen, do not activate these particular neurons in the monkey.

Following the initial discovery, the Rizzolatti lab showed that mirror neurons can be sensitive to very small differences between two

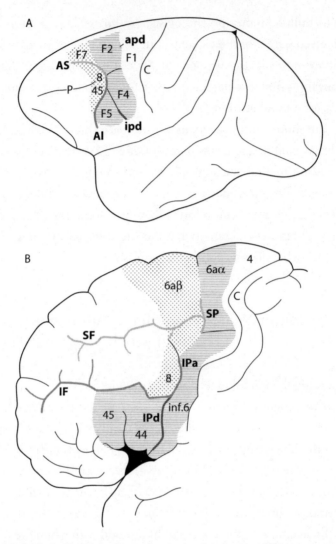

Figure 6.2. A (Top): Drawing of a monkey brain, showing area F5 in premotor cortex where mirror neurons were first found. F1 is the primary motor area. F2, F4 and F5 are premotor areas anterior to the motor strip; AS arcuate sulcus. B (Bottom): Drawing of the frontal region of the human brain showing area 44 (part of the inferior frontal gyrus), the area believed to be homologous to F5 and, along with area 45, also known in the human brain as Broca's area. The shading represents areas with anatomical and functional homologies. IF: inferior frontal sulcus; SF: superior frontal sulcus; IPa: inferior precentral sulcus; SP: superior precentral sulcus. The other numbers refer to Brodmann numbering of areas. Reprinted from G. Rizzolatti and M. Arbib, "Language within Our Grasp," *Trends in Neurosciences* 21 (1998):188–94. With permission from Elsevier.

similar observed actions.[42] Some neurons respond differentially to observations of grasping-to-get versus grasping-to-eat, even when the two movements are kinetically very similar. For example, a subset of neurons respond when the monkey either sees or makes a reaching movement where the object grasped is placed in a container on one's shoulder, but a different population of neurons respond when he sees or makes a very similar movement that grasps an object and brings it to the mouth.[43] In their reports, the Rizzolatti lab interpreted these data as showing that these neurons code for *action understanding*, by which they meant that the neurons represent a *goal* or *intention*. Not surprisingly, this claim caused a commotion because it implies a link between mirror neurons and the attribution of mental states—or at least one mental state, namely intention. Accordingly, it raised the possibility that the discovery of mirror neurons might open a door to understanding the neurobiology of mental attribution more generally.[44] A wonderfully exciting prospect, to be sure.

Inspired by the idea that mirror neurons might code for intentions, a more ambitious hypothesis took hold: perhaps a mirror neuron system might explain having a "theory of mind," whereby not only can I attribute to you a goal, but also fears, desires, feelings, and beliefs. The idea that an explanation for "mind reading" all but falls out of the discovery of mirror neurons was surprisingly popular among cognitive scientists almost immediately. People took up mirror neurons as though the connection to mental attributions was essentially self-explanatory, or very nearly so. In 1998, neuroscientist Vittorio Gallese and philosopher Alvin Goldman proposed that mirror neurons support the detection of mental states of others through a process of *simulation*. Thus they offered a general hypothesis to explain mental attribution operations in terms of mirror neuron function.[45] Fine, but how does the brain perform a simulation yielding those results?

The way attribution via simulation is supposed to work is that when I see you make a certain movement, such as grasping to eat, neurons in my premotor cortex *simulate* that movement, sort of matching the movement but without actually making the movement. If the resulting neuronal activity matches the activity that typically occurs when I intend to grasp for food, then I know what you intend to do. Since I know what that movement means in *my simulation* (I intend to eat), I just infer that it means the same thing for you—*you* intend to eat. As it was explained, "Because the monkey knows the outcome of the motor act it executes, it recognizes the goal of the motor act done by another individual when this act triggers the same set of neurons that are active during the execution of that act."[46] The proposed mechanism is meant to explain only the attribution of intentions or goals, not the further question of how attribution of beliefs or emotions is supposed to work. Altogether, it was a package that seemed highly promising.

Intriguing as the simulation proposal was, at the time it was largely speculative, and reached well beyond the data from monkeys showing merely that a subset of neurons were active in both execution and observation of grasping of objects. As neuroscientists were quick to complain, the available data did not rule out the more humdrum, but by no means uninteresting, hypothesis that the coding of movements by mirror neurons can be very fine-grained, and hence they distinguish between grasping-to-get and grasping-to-eat. This suggests that perhaps the data could be understood without the more obscure hypothesis of simulation, a hypothesis beset by problems of its own, as we are about to see. The monkeys in the Parma lab had been exposed to many instances of grasping food or grasping tools, as well as observing themselves grasping food and tools, and to the cautious, it seems likely that these relationships were associated through exposure. So far as the data are concerned, such multimodal neurons (responding to both seeing and doing) are probably just . . . well, just multimodal neurons. If so, their response properties are the outcome of sensory and motor convergence, coding for associations between the monkey observing his own hand and executing a movement, and then generalizing in a context-sensitive way.[47] Mental attribution in the full sense (whatever exactly that is) may not be part of what is going on at all.[48]

(This comment in no way denigrates associative learning as "mere association," since it can be very rich in its effects.)

The hypothesis that simulation is involved in intention attribution needed to be fleshed out by an account of the mechanism to explain how it worked. In 2005, an important paper from the Rizzolatti lab asserted, "This mechanism for understanding intention appears to be rather simple. Depending on which motor chain is activated, the observer is going to have an internal representation of what, most likely, the action agent is going to do. What is more complex is to specify how the selection of a particular chain occurs. After all, what the observer sees is just a hand grasping a piece of food or an object."[49] Boiled down, the simulation theory says the brain process for attributing an intention to another person involves three steps: (1) the observed movement is matched with activation in my own motor system; (2) the intention that goes with that particular movement, in my own case will then automatically be represented and so made known to me; (3) I attribute that same intention to the observed person.[50]

Three interlaced problems face the three steps: How is the selection of a matching motor chain accomplished by the brain? How, by observing and then simulating your movement, does my brain come to represent what my own intention would be in making the movement you made? And how does the brain decide what is the relevant intention of the observed individual from simulation of a movement? As Fogassi admitted in the 2005 paper, from movement alone, one may not be able to tell much about the intention of the observed individual, though he does not dwell on how difficult the problem actually is. But it is not a mere loose end; it is the fire in the tunnel.

Suppose I see an individual make an arm movement. Is he waving at me or signaling to his pals? Is he just stretching or wanting to ask a question? Is he trying to confuse me or does he even see me at all? As we saw in discussing mental attribution, associations between movements and outcomes are not sufficient to get very far in answering normal questions about intentions. One needs to know a lot more:

what the observed person probably thinks and knows and wants, for example. So if my brain merely simulates the hand raising, I still don't have a clue what your intention is.

To address—the first puzzle—how the brain figures out which "motor chain" is the one to match during observation and hence perform the simulation—Erhan Oztop, Mitsuo Kawato, and Michael Arbib developed an artificial neural network model.[51] Using a standard training algorithm, their model learns first to make associations between execution and self-observation of a specific movement; then the network extends recognition to observation of movements of others. While it succeeds in modeling basic movements, the model is limited to "understanding" only basic actions of others, such as my raising my arm, as opposed to more complex actions, such as greeting or warning by raising my arm. Without diminishing their modeling achievement, we can see that behind the vast majority of simple actions is a *higher level* intention, where the simple action is but a means to a complex end. Thus, to emphasize the point, I may raise my arm, motivated by any number of completely different intentions: to ask the teacher a question or signal the soldiers to charge or reveal my position to my hunting group or to stretch out my shoulder muscles or to vote for building a school, and so on and on.[52] I cannot remember the last time I raised my arm with no intention other than to raise my arm; maybe in the crib. Merely mirroring a movement will not tap into the range of higher-order intentions, or select the right one, for which a lot of background understanding, probably including a theory of mind, is needed.

Another limitation with the neural network model in its current form is that attributing an intention to the action requires that the observer has performed that action himself. Can we understand hitherto unperformed actions (can the appropriate intention be attributed)? Often, yes. If I have observed a cow being milked on at least one occasion, I can recognize quite well on a new occasion the intention behind tying up the cow, getting the milking stool, and putting the milk pail under the cow's bag—even if I have never milked a cow myself. (This seems to be true also of my dog, who is quite unable to milk a cow.) Moreover, even if I have never *seen* a camel milked, I will quickly recognize what is going on by analogy with my background knowledge of cow-milking. Ditto for a million other actions we can understand—pulling teeth, preparing a body for burial, amputating a leg, setting a bone, harpooning a seal . . . and so on. I may even understand an action I have neither previously executed nor previously observed, such as skinning a rabbit, skidding logs, or traveling on a zipline or a hang glider.

If we consider the attribution of intentions only in an artificially restricted domain, for example attributing basic motor intentions involving very familiar actions that the observer has previously and frequently performed himself, then the Oztop, Kawato, and Arbib model looks like progress. But as soon as we contemplate the richness of intentions in everyday life, the progress, while quite possibly on the right track, looks limited.[53] The question is whether the model gets us to the right first step, or whether it is a misstep.

The point is, without some magic, my brain's simulation of your movement is not likely to result in either my or your intention coming to be represented in my brain. Ironically, what does appear likely is that if we are able to simulate others in our imagination, that is partly because we already have skills that come with a theory of mind. Going in the other direction—explaining those skills merely in terms of simulation of movements—looks unpromising.

Criticism, it might be protested, is very well, but do I have a better theory of those social skills, of how they are acquired and developed? No, alas, but I am disinclined to be deflected from the search for a good theory by investing in an approach that seems to have an uncertain future.

Attributing an intention to another's arm-raising movement (e.g., he intends to ask a question) is supposed to depend upon the observer's brain representing what the observer's intention would be were she to make that movement. *Self*-attribution of intention (step 2) was supposed to be the easy part of the simulation story. Behind the seeming simplicity referred to in the 2005 Rizzolatti paper (when a chain of motor commands is activated in the observer, *the observer knows what he would be intending*) there is a huge, and largely unknown, neural complexity supporting "self-knowledge."[54] It is anything but obvious how, in neural terms, I can be aware of what I intend or believe or desire or feel. Think of it this way: how is activity in premotor neurons represented by other neurons as correlating with a specific intention, such as an intention to apologize as opposed to an intention to insult? A neuron, though computationally complex, is just a neuron. It is not an intelligent homunculus. If a neural network represents something complex, such as the intention to insult, it must have the right input and be in the right place in the neural circuitry to do that. [55]

Relying on introspection, Descartes concluded that the particulars of one's own mental states are "transparent" or "given"; they are self-evident, plain and simple. Hence which mental state *is occurring* and what it is *about* (e.g., a belief about Queen Elizabeth's corgis as opposed to a thought about how to open an oyster) does not need any explanation. According to the Cartesian, being self-revealing is just the way the processes in the nonphysical soul *are*. From a neuroscience perspective, however, we know all too well that self-attribution of mental states must be supported by complex computational (information processing) and representational mechanisms. Of these mechanisms, we know almost nothing.

That computational mechanisms must underlie normal self-attribution is dramatically evident from pathological cases, such as split-brain subjects in whom the two hemispheres have been separated surgically as part of the treatment of intractable epilepsy. This was done by cutting the corpus callosum, which is a sheet of nerves connecting the right and left hemispheres across the midline. The surgery is called a commissurotomy, and its effect is to disrupt communication between right and left hemispheres. In these subjects, purposeful behavior may be exhibited by the left hand, for example in response to a command sent by the experimenter only to the right hemisphere ("close the door"). Owing to the sectioning of the corpus callosum, the cortex of the left hemisphere (which is dominant for speech) has no access to a representation of the intention formed in the right; it knows nothing about the command sent by the experimenter. As neuroscientist Michael Gazzaniga observed, the left hemisphere, when queried about the action, effortlessly confabulates ("I closed the door because there was a cool breeze coming in").[56] It is not just that that the left hemisphere lacks access to the premotor activity of the right, it also lacks access to the motivating circumstance—to the command received only by the right, to the desire to respond to the command, and who knows what else—though it does have full access to the visual observation of the whole body movement. The point here then is that knowing one's own intention is not self-evident in some magical sense, but requires elaborate organization of information.

Alien hand syndrome is another example demonstrating the complexity behind self-knowledge of intentions and motivations. In this neurological condition, damage to the anterior commissure (another, smaller, communicating sheet between the left and right hemispheres) or the corpus callosum may result in one hand executing actions of which the person—or at least the left hemisphere—has no awareness. On occasion the left and right hands may engage in competing actions (e.g., one hand picks up the phone, the other puts it back), or one hand may begin a task such as making toast, while the other begins to make porridge. More extremely, one of the patient's hands may even try to choke her, while the other attempts to pull the choking hand off her throat. In these cases, each motivating intention seem confined to a single hemisphere, and hence opposing actions by the two hands, guided by distinct intentions, can occur.

The self-evidence of my knowledge of my intentions is a surface feature of introspection, part of the brain's self-model that masks a lot of messy neural details from inner inspection. To make matters more complicated, some allegedly self-evident truths about mental states are actually false. You might suppose it is self-evident that at any given moment, the clarity (area of fine resolution) of your visual perception is roughly the size of the laptop screen in front of you. As every psychology major is shocked to learn, however, in fact at any given 300-millisecond interval, the area of high-resolution perception is only about the size of the tip of your thumb at arm's length. Your eyes make a *saccadic shift* (a little change in focal direction) about three times each second, and your brain integrates over time the signals received by the retina to create the highly useful and compelling illusion of laptop-sized clarity at any given moment. Taking this caution to heart, we might wonder how much of what seems to be self-evident knowledge of our own intentions is also more iffy than certain.

Additionally, doubts about the accuracy and precision of self-knowledge of intentions are supported by careful experiments by social psychologists.[57] Surprisingly perhaps, the data indicate that in the course of business-as-usual decision-making, our intentions are not quite as specific and concrete as we report them to have been after the fact.[58] Rather, in some cases, the detailed specificity seems to emerge only when we are called upon to explain what we did: why we chose A rather than B. For example, in an experiment conducted in a shopping mall, passers-by were given the chance to taste two kinds of unlabeled jams, and then choose the one they preferred, which they would be given for free. After they made their choice, say apricot, the experimenter, in fussing around to supposedly give them the chosen jam, switched the jars, and gave them the jam not chosen—say blueberry. They were then asked to taste again, and verify their choice, *which they most often did*, not commenting on the switch. When asked to explain their choice, they said such things as that blueberry (the one *not* chosen, but received) had always been their favorite, that they liked the rich flavor, and so on. They seem not to have noticed the switch, and were amazed if the switch was pointed out. Of course choosing free jars of jam is not greatly consequential, so it may be that for many choices where it matters little, the intention is nothing like as specific as in more consequential cases.[59]

In skilled behavior, such as hockey or cooking, many aspects of decision-making are grounded in habit, and hence are automatic. A hockey player can explain, when interviewed later, why he passed to a teammate rather than taking the shot himself, but probably no such a well-formed conscious intention played an actual role in the neural activity that produced the behavior. There was pattern recognition followed by a skilled movement, but no deliberation.

Finally, in considering how we develop the capacity to self-attribute, it is most likely that the attribution of intentions and goals is not first grounded in awareness of one's own case and *then* extended to others; rather, self-attribution and other-attribution are probably co-learned.[60] As a side note, psychologists Roy Baumeister and E. J. Masicampo argue that conscious thought is an adaptation that emerges from pressure for sophisticated social and cultural interactions, including the simulation of possible plan outcomes—how others might feel, respond, and react—and in humans, the simulation of speech.[61] This is a rather appealing idea, relative to the earlier discussions concerning the representational efficiencies achieved by the attribution of mental states.

Humans, Intentions, and Mirror Neurons

So far, our discussion of evidence for mirror neurons has been confined to monkeys. The supposition that mirror neurons are also behind our human capacity to attribute goals and intentions to others is based on the reasonable idea that human brains are organized similarly to monkey brains. Are there areas in the human brain that show "mirroring," in the sense that neurons in those regions respond both to the observation of another body performing a specific action and one's own execution of that same action?

For ethical reasons, recording from single neurons is not done for experimental purposes in humans, so there is almost no direct evidence.[62] Nevertheless, imaging techniques such as positron emission tomography (PET) or functional magnetic resonance imaging (fMRI) may be able to provide indirect evidence. Evidence for classical mirroring in humans would be a demonstration of increased activity in an area of the brain that is homologous to the monkey's F5 or inferior frontal gyrus, under conditions both of observing an action and executing it. Even if this is successfully demonstrated, it cannot show that an *individual neuron* responds in both conditions, as the single-cell data do in the monkeys, but it will at least provide significant support for mirroring.

Although there is a long-standing conviction among cognitive neuroscientists that mirroring of the kind described has been well established in humans, in fact the case for mirroring in humans is still somewhat contentious. The contention is partly owed to assorted difficulties associated with analyzing fMRI data, such as averaging results across a group of individuals, which can obscure the question of whether each subject showed the required overlap in a specific area.[63] There have also been differences in experimental protocol used by different labs that make comparisons confusing.

Finally, in 2009 neuroscientists Valeria Gazzola and Christian Keysers undertook a study in which they analyzed fMRI data for subjects taken singly, as opposed to averaging across individuals, and testing precisely whether there was increased activity in both the observation and execution conditions. In all sixteen subjects, they did find increased activity in particular voxels in area 44 (believed to be homologous to monkey F5) and the inferior parietal cortex, during both observation and execution. In my skeptical judgment, this was the first really convincing data to support coactivation in humans of area 44 (part of the inferior frontal gyrus or IFG) and inferior parietal areas in a way that approximates what was found in monkeys at the level of single cells.[64] Of course the data do not answer the further interpretive and causal questions.[65] Interestingly, their data revealed many additional areas whose activity also increased: dorsal premotor, supplementary motor, middle cingulate, somatosensory, superior parietal, middle temporal cortex, and cerebellum. This is a *lot* of brain landscape, and extends well beyond the "classic" mirror neuron areas described in the monkey experiments.[66] Further complicating the story for the mirror system proponents, Rebecca Saxe found correlations between mental state attribution and yet other areas: the temporal parietal junction, especially on the right, and also the mPFC.[67]

Additional misgivings come from other labs using fMRI that have reported results that strongly implicate the mPFC in the representation of one's own intentions, not area 44 (the classical mirror neuron system).[68] In one experimental protocol, subjects in the scanner were asked to choose one of two actions to perform — either adding or subtracting two numbers — and to hold the specific intention in mind during an unpredictable delay (between about 3 and 11 seconds) until the two numbers were presented. The spatial pattern of activity in the medial frontal pole was different depending on whether subjects were intending to add or subtract when the numbers eventually appeared. If knowing one's intention involves the brain representing that intention, it looks like the more posterior areas such as area 44 may be less important that the anterior areas of the PFC (see figure 6.3). The simulation theory implies that if these areas are involved in self-knowledge of intention, they should also be involved in simulating another's intention. Various hunches could be trotted out here, but the central questions remain unanswered: what are the mechanisms involved in mental attribution to self and others, and how important, if at all, is simulation in carrying out those functions?

Mirroring and Empathy

Granting that there is still only weak evidence that a mirror neuron system is the substrate for the ability to attribute intentions to others,

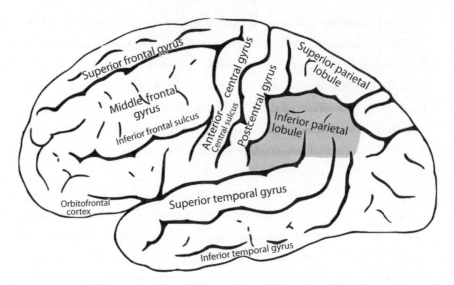

Figure 6.3. Diagram of the left hemisphere of the human brain showing the location of major sulci and gyri, and the inferior parietal lobule (in gray). Based on Wikimedia Commons, public domain. (http://commons.wikimedia.org/w/index.php?title= Special%3ASearch&search=inferior+parietal)

many researchers believe that our empathic responses present a better case for simulation as the means by which we identify the mental states of others.[69] My having empathy for your predicament, according to this view, depends on simulating, in my brain, your sad facial expression. This action makes me feel a little sad, and thus I can recognize what you are experiencing. Ditto for fear, disgust, anger, and so forth. Taking this fairly old idea and packaging it in terms of mirror neurons, neuroscientist Marco Iacoboni has proposed a general account for empathy according to which "the core imitation circuitry would simulate (or internally imitate) the facial emotional expressions of other people. This activity would then modulate activity in the limbic system (through the insula) where the emotion associated with a given facial expression is felt by the observer."[70] As Iacoboni sums up the hypothesis, mimicry precedes the recognition of what you are feeling, and gives us the basis for ascribing a feeling to you.[71]

It is well known that seeing another's misery often makes us feel miserable ourselves, and that our spirits are often lifted by observing someone else's joy. So much is not news. Iacoboni is arguing for the further point that recognition of another's misery requires mimicry via "core imitation circuitry." What is the evidence for this specific claim?

Consider first the correlational data; then we can consider causality. In a landmark study, Bruno Wicker and colleagues[72] scanned subjects in the fMRI while the subjects viewed a face that looked disgusted, and also when subjects got a strong whiff of a disgusting smell. The changes in brain activity were in the same general location—the inferior frontal operculum (opercular "taste cortex") and the adjacent anterior insula, both known to be sensitive to disgusting tastes (see figure 3.5).

For pain, there happen to be some human data on single neurons recorded during cingulate surgery for refractory psychiatric conditions. W. D. Hutchison and colleagues recorded from single cells in the anterior cingulate cortex (ACC) during cingulotomy, and found several cells in three subjects that responded both to a painful stimulus, and to the observation of a painful stimulus applied to another person. They reported that the cells' response to observed pain was less than the response to the subject's own pain, and suggested that the response in the observation condition might be an *anticipation* of a painful stimulus applied to the subject himself.[73] The report does not address the matter of the causal role of such cells in attributing pain states to other people. A number of labs using fMRI have found coactivation of ACC and anterior insula, both when subjects are given a painful stimulus, and when they are shown someone else grimacing with pain during application of acupuncture needles. Some labs also saw activity in the somatosensory cortex (processing touch, pressure, vibration and so forth; see figure 3.4, page 38) in both feeling and observing conditions.[74] Moreover, there was a correlation between the intensity of the pain—either felt or observed—and the level of activity in the somatosensory areas.[75] Further, differences in activity levels in the ACC are seen depending on whether the observed recipient of pain is a loved one (high) or a stranger (lower).[76]

Psychologists have used behavioral techniques to investigate whether the motor system has a role in the simulation of feelings. For example, when experimenters ask subjects to perform a simple facial mimicry task while observing a face expressing an emotion, the observation interferes with the motor task.[77] In other studies, it was found that biting on a pencil interfered with a subject's recognition of happy faces more than those expressing fear, disgust, or sadness. This finding is in line with the observation that expressions of happiness generate the greatest facial action, and suggests that recognition of emotional expressions may be differentially sensitive to simulation.[78] Nevertheless, people with paralyzed faces can recognize facial expressions of emotions, so the role of the motor system in recognizing emotions is still not clearly understood.

One of the more careful fMRI experiments to test the correlation of activity during seen and felt pain was done by neuroscientists India Morrison and Paul Downing.[79] Analyzed at the group level, the data indicated coactivation in a small region of the anterior cingulate cortex and the anterior insula. This overlap seems to support mirroring. Recognizing that group averaging may mask important differences between individual subjects, they reanalyzed the data, looking at individual subjects. Then a rather different picture emerged. In six of eleven subjects, there was a small area active in both the observing and feeling conditions; in the remaining five, however, the areas activated by seen and felt pain did *not* overlap. In all subjects, activations levels differed depending on whether the pain was seen or felt, consistent with the data from Hutchinson and colleagues. The Morrison and Downing results raise the level of uncertainty concerning analysis of fMRI data more generally, and in particular, whether coactivation of neurons during observed and felt sensations or emotions is necessary for empathy.

So what about causality and mechanism? The case for simulation, as characterized by Iacoboni,[80] has not yet been established in my view.[81] Here is the kind of puzzle that complicates a simple causal connection: animal and human studies suggest that fear processing is strongly associated with the amygdala, and textbooks routinely claim that feelings of fear emerge from activity in amygdala circuitry. Nevertheless, three patients who, through a rare disease, suffered a loss of the amygdala on both sides of the brain, have normal recognition of fearful faces and can display fear in social situations.[82] The lesions all occurred in adulthood, so it is not known whether a different pattern would exist for someone with early-onset amygdala lesions could recognize fear in others. What is clear is that patients with frontotemporal dementia and whose insular cortex is damaged tend not to feel empathy, or to feel intense emotions themselves.[83] The insula plays an important role in feeling social pain and distress, but so far has not been directly linked to mirror neurons. Though these observations do not disconfirm the simulation hypothesis, they do highlight the need for that hypothesis to take account of them in some systematic fashion.

Perhaps it would be salutary at this stage to loose the skeptical hounds on the whole claim that empathy depends on simulation, in order to see where that leads us. So, mindful of the flaws, I will start with myself. What exactly *do* I feel if I see someone crying after being stung on the foot by a wasp (and I know what that feels like)? There is a lot of variability as a function of context, for example depending on who got stung (my baby or an intruder). Here is my phenomenology, for what it is worth: when I saw my granddaughter and my husband stung on the legs by wasps, I did not literally feel a sting, and I did not feel anything even vaguely painful in my legs. It should be noted that "touch synesthetes"—about 1% of the population—do claim to literally feel the same touch in the same place as the person observed, and do have activation in lower as well as higher somatosensory areas when observing others being touched.[84] What I did feel was a visceral, generalized sense of awfulness (that homeostatic emotion Bud Craig investigates), and the urge to apply antihistamines, or, failing that, mud. More exactly (or perhaps less exactly), I would say I felt so sorry for them. Moreover, though *you* will have a different feeling depending on whether you were burned or stung or cut, *my* awfulness response seems to be more or less the same for each of your mishaps. That synesthetes are such a tiny fraction of the population suggests that the rest of us usually respond with only generalized feelings of awfulness when seeing someone yelping from a recent wasp sting. Additionally, the sensory anatomy of synesthetes is a little different.

Further skeptical questions shoulder in for attention. Observing that someone is angry may not produce anger in the observer, but fear or embarrassment or, depending on the situation, possibly even laughter. I may recognize that someone is grieving or feeling annoyed without grieving or feeling annoyed myself. I may recognize that someone is disappointed without feeling disappointed myself. If it is my enemy who is in pain, I may feel not pain, but relief (related to *schadenfreude*, which may not be a morally worthy response, but is very common nonetheless). If I see a colleague look disgusted when I make a proposal in a department meeting, I am apt to feel either annoyed or amused, but not disgusted. These sorts of difficulties with the simulation theory of mental attribution have long been appreciated, and the current excitement over mirror neurons does nothing to put them to rest.

Goldman confronts these difficulties by conceding that mechanisms other than simulation can be used to attribute mental states. Nevertheless, he does maintain that simulation is the fundamental process.[85] While this could be correct, the concession could be just a convenient means for explaining away countervailing results by invoking unknown "other mechanisms," even while the case for simulation as fundamental causal requirement in mental attribution has yet to be made solid.

A different, and arguably more powerful, hypothesis regarding the mechanisms underlying compassion is that the empathic responses are an extension of the feeling of awfulness that arises in mammals when our infants are distressed or separated from us, and when they make distress calls.[86] If, as hypothesized, in humans the care circle has been extended to include care for mates, kin, and kith, then compassion for mates, kin, and kith may not require special simulation mechanisms, though the capacity to imagine and evaluate future consequences of a plan may be extended to imagining many other things. This approach also is consistent with the fact that by and large, people show a more intense response to another's misery, depending on the closeness of the relationship to the injured. Parents, for example, are more acutely sensitive to the miseries of their offspring than to the miseries of strangers.[87]

Developmental psychologists have proposed that the infant seems to have an innate disposition to be drawn to, or attentive to, biological movements that are "like me," in some very rudimentary sense.[88] This is a kind of platform, which can develop into an increasingly sophisticated framework, as the child gains experience of his own body and feelings, and interacts with others. In some manner, poorly understood at the neural level, the "like me" framework becomes increasingly richer—with the self-attributions and the other-attributions probably coevolving. Neuroscientist Gyorgi Buzsáki makes the point this way: "The brain gradually acquires its self-awareness by learning to predict the neuronal performance of other brains. . . . [T]he acquisition of self-consciousness requires the feedback from other brains."[89] Understanding the neurobiological mechanisms underlying these kinds of social skills, such as gaze following, mental attribution, and empathy, is a continuing challenge. To the cautious, it is evident that much remains to be discovered.

Imitation and "Mirror Neurons"

It might seem obvious that imitation is closely linked to mirroring goals and movements, and hence to a "mirror neuron system." Iacoboni, quoted earlier, refers to a "core imitation circuitry" that he believes is deployed in empathy.[90] Here again, a close, critical look at the data suggest a need for caution concerning what has actually been established about circuitry supporting imitation.

First, mirroring as described in the classical experiments with monkeys is not imitation: the monkey does not imitate what he sees, nor do his muscles show incipient movement. Second, though area 44 (in the IFG) is frequently assumed to correspond to area F5 in the macaque, a recent meta-analysis showed that there is no solid evidence that area 44 is involved during imitation.[91] Other areas, however, did show increased activity, including the premotor area 6, area 7 (parietal cortex), and area 40 (superior temporal). Even the motor strip, area 4, was modestly more active than area 44. To be clear, the meta-analysis does not demonstrate that no "mirror neuron system" is involved in human imitation. What it does show is only that the presumptive claim that area 44 is a part of the human mirror neuron system, and hence is part of the core circuitry for imitation, is not consistent with the fMRI data showing which areas have increased activity during imitation. The long and short of it is that we do not really know how imitative behavior is produced.[92] Eventually the pathways and mechanisms will be identified, but we are not there yet.

Theory of Mind, Autism, and Mirror Neurons

Individuals diagnosed with autism are likely to show withdrawal from social interaction, sleep disorders, poor understanding of others' behavior, weak communicative skills, lack of empathy, and perseverative behavior (not adapting behavior to changes in conditions).[93] Many show retardation, about 25% have seizures, some learn language, but others do not. Variations in severity of the symptoms have prompted a revision of the diagnosis "autism" to "autism spectrum disorder," or ASD.

In contrast to those with Down syndrome, subjects with ASD tend not to make eye contact, are not cuddly, jolly, or apt to engage spontaneously in social interactions. Of particular interest for this chapter, they typically show impairments in imitation.[94] The baffling nature of the etiology of the disease, along with its terrible cost in human suffering, has motivated researchers to search for explanations in terms of brain abnormalities. As John Hughes ruefully commented in his recent review, nearly every conceivable etiology has been mentioned to explain this serious disorder.[95]

No consistent structural abnormality in the brain has been seen so far, so the hunch is that the salient differences probably exist at the microstructural level, and will perhaps be revealed physiologically using methods such as fMRI and EEG. Since subjects with ASD have deficits in attributing mental states,[96] researchers wondered whether there might be a mirror neuron system abnormality that could explain the deficits.

Some studies have shown behavioral differences between ASD subjects and healthy controls during spontaneous imitation. For example, one study presented ASD participants and typical controls with photographs of clearly happy and clearly angry faces.[97] Participants' responses to these photographs were measured with sensors placed over facial muscles responsible for smiling and frowning. Typical participants quickly responded to the presentation of happy faces by smiling and angry faces by frowning. However, the faces of ASD participants remained flat, showing no spontaneous mirroring of the expressions. Importantly, this was not because ASD participants failed to recognize happiness or anger, or did not know how to smile or frown. When the researchers explicitly asked ASD participants to "make the faces like the ones on the screen," their facial responses were fully appropriate and indistinguishable from the typical group. Other studies using other stimuli and designs reported similar findings suggesting that it is harder (though not always impossible) to spontaneously trigger the imitative process in autism.[98] Supporting the "mirror neuron" explanation of such behavioral differences, one fMRI study observed lower activation in the area 44 (among other areas) when ASD children viewed emotional facial expressions.[99]

A key measure supposedly linked to activity in the mirror neurons system is a change in a μ-waveform (μ-suppression), detected by EEG during performance and observation. Some researchers have reported seeing differences between ASD subjects and healthy controls.[100] Further studies indicate that μ-suppression turns out to be the same in both high-functioning ASD subjects and healthy controls, hence disconfirming the hypothesis that μ-suppression is an index of mirror neuron activity; alternately, if it is such an index, then disconfirming the hypothesis that mirror neuron activity is abnormal in ASD subjects. Which alternative obtains is not settled. Subjects with ASD differ greatly in intelligence, and a study using preadolescent high-functioning subjects with ASD may give different results from one that includes a range of IQs and ages.[101] Disappointing though it may be, the most we can say about the autism–mirror neuron link is that further study is needed. In the meanwhile, yet again, caution seems to be the order of the day.

Imitation, Unconscious Mimicry, and Social Capacities

Because the emergence of highly developed cultural traditions among humans has been associated with the human capacity and inclination to imitate,[102] there is one additional area I wish briefly to explore: unconscious mimicry. Psychological studies on unconscious mimicry in humans show that the posture, mannerisms, voice contours, and words of one subject are unknowingly mimicked by the other. Such mimicry most people do, regularly, as part of normal social interactions. In psychological experiments exploring this phenomenon, a student subject and an experimental assistant (not identified to the student as such, and not known to the student) are put in a room, where the cover story is that they are to work on a project, and observers record whether there is mimicking behavior as the interaction occurs. Subjects do typically mimic the assistant's movements, such as putting the chin on the hand, tapping a pencil, crossing legs, leaning back in the chair, and so forth. Subjects are not aware of their mimicry, and hence the label *unconscious* mimicry. In a further test, the assistants are given instructions either to mimic the subjects they are working with, or to inhibit any mimicry. Subjects whom the assistant (knowingly) mimics subsequently tend to evaluate the assistant more favorably than if they were not mimicked.[103] Mimicked subjects also tend to be more helpful than those not mimicked. For example, when, as they leave, a box falls to the floor, scattering pencils, mimicked subjects are more likely to replace the pencils on the desk than subjects who were not mimicked. This suggests that unconscious mimicry has a significant role in affiliation, and in establishing a warm relationship. Incidentally, if you are at a social gathering, perhaps with various people new to you, and you try to inhibit your own mimicry, you will likely find it quite difficult. The normal tendency is to smile when they smile, laugh when they laugh, stand if they are standing, so forth.

Another manipulation consists in creating social stress in a subject before she enters the room to work with the assistant. This is done by having the subject play Cyberball on a computer, a game where a virtual ball is tossed between players, one of whom is the subject. Experimenters alter the game so that after a few minutes the ball is rarely passed to the subject. Remarkably, this virtual isolation yields sufficient social stress to produce an effect in subsequent mimicry. Subjects who are socially stressed in this manner tend to show greater mimicry in the experimental condition than subjects who are not socially stressed. It is almost as if the stressed subjects are trying extra hard (unconsciously) to win favor with the other person. The dominant hypothesis explaining the data from unconscious mimicry is that mimicry acts as social glue.[104] This does seem plausible, but I found myself puzzling about this question: *why* does mimicry function as social glue? Why do we feel more positive about people who mimic our low-level gestures, even when we are quite unaware of the mimicry? Why does the brain put a lot of effort, and hence a lot of energy, into mimicry, and what is the significance of the information it gets?

Probably we like mimicry at this low level because it shows that you are like me. Why should that matter? Because it enables me to predict your behavior a little better than if you are very *unlike* me. How does it enable such a prediction? The main part of the answer is likely that I am familiar with how I respond, so I can use that to predict how you, if similar to me, will likely respond. The related neural component that I suspect supports the story is this: imitation by the very young is an early sign of a normally developing frontal cortex, something needed in all mammals, but especially needed in all highly social mammals. The mother chimpanzee or rhesus or human need not be aware that it is such a sign. She needs only to respond to imitation as attractive in the young. Increased strength of attachment with imitation is the mother's implicit recognition that, frontally speaking, the infant is on a normal developmental track.

Imitative performance predicts that the baby has the neural where-withal to learn what he needs to learn to survive, particularly in the social world, but also in the wider world. More succinctly, a baby that can imitate probably has a normal social brain. Other things being equal, a normal social learning capacity is a good predictor that the child will thrive, and hence is worth further investment, to put it in biological terms. Mimicry signals the presence of a social capacity, namely the capacity to learn to predict what others will do and feel, the capacity to learn group practices, and the emotional capacity to behave appropriately. It also predicts that the child can pick up knowledge about how to get on in life—how to forage, defend, make shelters, and so on.[105] More darkly, if the infant fails in general to imitate, the failure is a predictor that things do not bode well for the child.[106] Though it would be hard to test, especially in the field, the hypothesis predicts that babies whose frontal organization fails to support early imitation may end up less well tended, perhaps with fewer resources, and hence may show failure to thrive.[107] Parents show great joy when the infant imitates, which probably increases their imitation of the infant, and the infant of them, and thus sets the infant on the royal road to social understanding.[108]

Thus, perhaps, the parent's delight in the infant's imitation. But whence our fondness for mimicry in later stages of life? The hypothesis connecting imitation to affiliative responses can be extended quite broadly, and I shall simplify to keep the main points from getting obscured: We like imitation in social situations (I laugh when you laugh, I eat the roast pig when you eat the roast pig, and so forth) because imitative behavior (not too much, just the right amount) is a powerful signal of social competence that allows me to predict that you are pretty much like me. Put simply, we like imitation because it tells us that your frontal brain is much like my frontal brain.

If you are not well known to me, it is reassuring for me if you behave as I do because then to some significant degree I can predict your behavior; you are *like me*. This means that I can predict, albeit roughly, what will make you aggressive, what you will be like around babies, whether you will reconcile after a tiff, whether you will reciprocate, and so forth. When I am reassured, my cortisol (stress hormone) levels fall, which means I feel less anxious, and that feels good. Additionally, feeling that someone is trustworthy is a positive, oxytocin-related, bonding emotion. Our mimicry of each other might also weakly imply that we will care enough to tend to our respective reputations in the normal way; that is, in a way that is conducive to group harmony and good citizenry. Roughly, "You are like me, and like my kin. They are okay, so you are probably okay too."

Oddball behavior, however, makes me anxious, because I cannot predict what you will do—whether you will be dangerous or nasty—and a dangerous or nasty person in our midst can cause a lot of pain. The possibility that you are dangerous raises my cortisol levels, as I have to be on guard and watchful, a state of my brain that is not pleasant for me.

As social sizing up develops over a few minutes, assuming I got the preliminary signals I needed, I may be motivated to reassure *you*. So I play my part in mimicry so that you do not start anxiously watching me, thereby making me uncomfortable, or excluding me, making me even more uncomfortable.[109] The general point, therefore, is that something roughly like this may be the background explanation for unconscious mimicry.

Here is a speculation concerning the advantages of unconscious mimicry in the social life of our ancestral hominins. Amalgamation of others into the group may serve to strengthen the manpower needed in defense and attack, or may add to the number of fertile females as well as diversify the gene pool. Nevertheless, amalgamation can be a risky business, and newcomers may undermine the welfare and harmony of the clan. There are many factors to be wary of, including the import of new diseases, but factors concerning sociality are crucial. That is, before accepting a new member, the clan will want assurance that newcomers are not cognitively or emotionally problematic. As a first-pass filter for trustworthiness and hence for a normal social brain, mimicry, albeit unconscious mimicry, serves passably well.

Suppose a stranger arrives at the home range. His conforming behavior suggests he has a normal social capacity, that he can acquire the local practices and is willing to do so. In a thousand different ways, his sociality is going to matter to those in the group. Moreover, if members of the kin group share certain mannerisms and social symbols, a newcomer may gain entry by showing that he/she is willing to expend energy to adopt the mannerisms and symbols. Successful imitative behavior gets one past the gate because it is a sign of social competence. It is not, to be sure, a fail-safe predictor, but it may be screen out those who are socially problematic. Certainly, full acceptance into the group is typically a fairly gradual affair. Hume noticed that we extend kindness more easily to those who are like us, who resemble us. His insight appears to be on the mark, and my hunch is that the explanation lies in the test for accepting newcomers as trustworthy group members.

To begin to test this hypothesis, psychologists asked subjects to view a video of two men interacting during an interview, and to assess the competence of both the interviewer and the applicant (both actually actors).[110] In one version of the video, the interviewer is a bit of an oaf and a boor, whereas in the second version he is gracious. The experiment also varied the behavior of the applicant: in one version, he does not reciprocate the interviewer's gestures, but in another he subtly mimics the gestures and body movements of the interviewer. Viewers are essentially oblivious to the mimicry at the conscious level. The surprising finding was that viewing subjects rated the applicant as less competent when he mimicked an oafish interviewer than when he mimicked a gracious one. Mimicking an oafish person, it seems, deserved an even lower rating than not mimicking at all. This suggests that mimicking a low-status or unworthy person is taken by others to be a sign of poor judgment on the part of the mimicker. That observers of mimicry judge others in this way suggests that individuals are highly sensitive not only to mimicry behavior in general, but to whom they should and should not mimic. This may also connect with findings in the social learning field showing that most subjects are likely to model themselves after successful rather than unsuccessful people, whatever the particular domain of activity where success is evident.[111] That these judgments are made by *observers* of social interactions indicates that there are many levels of social information in the social learning business.

• • •

The neurobiology of social skills, and in particular the nature of the capacity to attribute mental states to others, is a young but vigorous field. The coevolution of psychology and neuroscience will doubtless bring new knowledge along with many surprises to this area of research in the next decade. In the next chapter, I examine rules and norms: what is their place in moral behavior?

7. Not as a Rule

So far in this discussion, rules, norms, laws, and their ilk have been waiting in the wings, while values, learning, and motivated problem-solving have taken center stage. This is a consequence of the logic structuring this project, which acknowledges that although social problem-solving may in time *culminate* in explicit rules, antecedent and more basic are the *implicit* standards emerging from shared values—practices that most individuals pick up without much instruction but by imitation and observation.[1] For example, not offering to lend a hand in a circumstance where the offer could be construed as insulting is not explicitly formulated as a rule, and local standards do vary.[2] How much eye contact to have with a stranger, when laughing aloud is boorish, or when it ceases to be acceptable to charm the teacher, are likewise implicitly learned, and likewise vary across cultures. By contrast, laws that prohibit child labor in factories and mines, that restrict the power of the reigning monarch to raise taxes, or that use taxes to pay for a sewer system, are explicit, and emerge from the perception of misery resulting from the status quo, and from the collective recognition that things could be better given a different way of doing business.

For people eager for change from the current state, getting a vague *ideal* into a workable *law* often requires a major outlay in time and energy, and sometimes involves significant personal cost. Not surprisingly, unforeseen consequences of the new law may sour the heartfelt aspirations of those who had longed for social improvement, as with the law (1920–33) in the United States prohibiting the manufacture, import, transportation, and sale of alcoholic beverages.[3] By and large, explicit rules start with reflection on current practices, and depend on imagining how things could be different.[4] Success in getting a law into place will depend on a host of variables, and relies on the structure of the existing social organization. Over time, laws may undergo modification for many reasons, some that serve the interests of a powerful subgroup, some that serve the well-being of the group as a whole, some that reflect the psychiatric delusions of a manipulative despot.

Social wisdom, in Aristotle's view, depends on the early development of good habits, and the capacity to reason sensibly about specific social issues. It draws on complex skills, including the skill to deal effectively with social disorder and instabilities, to anticipate the consequences of a plan, and to foresee new problems, as well as the ability to negotiate productively about explicit rules and institutions. Good institutions, such as trial by jury rather than trial by ordeal, or institutions for regulating currency, have enormous impact on the well-being of individuals in social groups, and on how an individual's responses to social problem-solving are shaped. In Aristotle's view, at the core of living a worthy life is the goal of developing good institutions to provide a harmonious structure to the social lives of individuals living in a city or state.[5]

Putting Aristotle's prescient ideas into more contemporary form, we could say that for the most part, the brain's continuous decision-making business depends on a continuous process of settling into solutions to constraint satisfaction problems. A range of constraints provide value-tagged weights, and as the time for a decision is nigh, the networks settle into a minimum that roughly satisfies the constraints.[6] As the reward system responds to the pains and satisfactions of experience, social skills are acquired and habits formed.[7] Habits constitute a powerful constraint, representing, as they do, past solutions that worked well enough to become entrenched by the reward system, thereby economizing the constraint satisfaction process. Habits reflect social learning about what the group regards as right or wrong. Habits also reflect learning about the physical world. In selecting a path down a ski slope or the words to respond to a student's question, learned skills, recent experiences, and nonconscious evaluations of the circumstances are powerful and crucial constraints on choice of behavior.[8] The details of the nature of the neural processes that go into decision-making remain to be nailed down, but constitute some of the most relevant research for this book.

Distinguished moral philosophers are apt to complain that Aristotle is vague and wooly—that he fails to give specific principles telling us what is right and wrong. They may prefer instead the theory that *rules* are the essence of morality. Thus, "Morality is a set of fundamental rules that guide our actions," wrote the late Robert Solomon in his justly popular textbook, *Introducing Philosophy*.[9] John Rawls, arguably the most influential moral philosopher of the twentieth century, tried heroically to formulate the universal rules of fairness that ought to govern policy, legislation, and the development of institutions.[10] Legions of moral philosophers have spent their intellectual lives trying to make Rawls's approach work. In one of the deepest discussions of why the approach is flawed beyond redemption, philosopher Owen Flanagan sums up, "There is no such thing as universal ethical intuitions at the level Rawls was initially looking to locate them."[11] Philosopher Mark Johnson puts the point even more forcefully:

> I will suggest it is morally irresponsible to think and act as though we possess a universal, disembodied reason that generates absolute rules, decision-making procedures, and universal

or categorical laws by which we can tell right from wrong in any situation we encounter.[12]

My aim is not to scoff at well-meaning attempts to formulate good rules for our complex societies. Rather, my aim is to explain, albeit sketchily, how humans are able to evaluate a law as a bad law or a good law or a fair law, *without* appealing to a yet deeper law—something they actually do, and do regularly. Evaluation, as discussed, is rooted in the emotions and passions that are endemic to human nature, and in the social habits acquired through childhood. Evaluative processes exploit memory and draw upon the capacity for solving problems. Reason does not create values, but shapes itself around them and takes them in new directions.[13]

This chapter will take a close, and skeptical, look at the commonplace view that rules, and their conscious, rational application, are definitive of morality. A first preliminary point is that *if* rules are definitive of morality, and rules require language, then by definition, verbal humans are the only organisms with morality. This seems an unnecessarily restrictive conclusion, given the caring behavior of some highly social nonhuman animals.[14]

A second preliminary point is that the favorite rules often recited as central to morality regularly conflict with other favorite rules: "Charity begins at home" regularly conflicts with "Love your neighbor as yourself"; "Lying is wrong" can conflict with "Unkindness is wrong." "Honor your parents" may conflict with "Never aid and abet a murderer." Each of these rules has limitations, recognition of which is often implicit. To illustrate, a prototypical rule that people cite is "Killing is wrong." Yet most firmly believe that killing is acceptable in war, though even in war, sometimes it is wrong to kill—for example, one does not kill prisoners of war, and one does not kill noncombatants, though even on this topic, there are different views about whether killing noncombatants is wrong if they voluntarily act as human shields for the enemy . . . the qualifications and what-ifs pile on and on without end.

Interestingly, former Supreme Court Justice David Souter made the same point regarding flexibility with respect to the provisions of the American Constitution. As he noted, the First Amendment, according to which "Congress shall make no law . . . abridging the freedom of speech, or of the press," is not absolute; it can, and did, conflict with the government's responsibility for order and the security of the nation. The particular conflict he discusses concerns the case of the Pentagon Papers, which the *New York Times* and the *Washington Post* wished to publish, while the government wanted to suppress publication on grounds of national interest. As Souter explained:

> A choice may have to be made, not because language is vague but because the Constitution embodies the desire of the American people, like most people, to have things both ways. We want order and security, and we want liberty. And we want not only liberty but equality as well. These paired desires of ours can clash, and when they do a court is forced to choose between them, between one constitutional good and another one. The court has to decide which of our approved desires has the better claim, right here, right now, and a court has to do more than read fairly when it makes this kind of choice.[15]

The ability to appreciate when a circumstance is a fair exception, or which rule to follow when rules conflict, embodies some of the most refined aspects of social understanding. Going through life, we all acquire a lot of subtle, and often inarticulable, knowledge through our experiences—stories, examples, and observation. Gossip often relates tales of plans gone wrong, of avoidable disaster, of self-indulgence causing misery, of hypocrisy collapsing someone's position on the moral high ground. Exceptions to rules have special poignancy, as when the Unabomber's brother sorrowfully turned him in, or when obstetrician Henry Morgentaler stood up against the anti-abortion conventions in Canada, and after going to jail, saw new laws written, or when Galileo grimly retracted his claim that the sun was the center of the known universe in order to avoid torture by the Catholic Church. Thus adults who are doggedly insensitive to reasonable exceptions are said to lack common sense, and are roundly pilloried in stories such as the fool who refused to lie to a delusional schizophrenic wielding an assault rifle. In general, apart from baroque legislation like the income tax code, what counts as a reasonable exception to a rule is not itself determined by yet another, deeper rule specifying allowable exceptions to the rule, and so on down. Instead, exceptions are often determined by fair-minded, sensible judgment, whatever exactly that is. But whatever it is, the development of good habits seems to be important for it. Of which, more below.

Moral theories that leave room for exceptions to rules have tended to seem incomplete. Consequently, the awkwardness of dealing with exceptions to rough-and-ready rules (e.g., "Always tell the truth") has motivated many moral philosophers to search for universally applicable, *exceptionless* rules. Such rules are supposed to apply to everyone, under all circumstances, regardless of situational contingencies.

The Golden Rule ("Do unto others as you would have them do unto you") is very often held up as a judicious rule, an exceptionless rule, and a rule that is universally espoused, or very close to it. (Ironically perhaps, Confucius, though known to prefer the development of virtues to instruction by rules, might have been among the first to give voice to a version of this maxim, though given his broad approach to morality, it is likely he offered it as general advice rather than as an exceptionless rule.[16]) So it must asked: since we are familiar with the Golden Rule, and it seems like an excellent rule, why are moral philosophers still hunting around for the fundamental rule that should guide all behavior? What more than adherence to the Golden Rule do we need to live a virtuous life?

The general appeal of the Golden Rule has not gone unappreciated by moral philosophers, but they have also realized it has shortcomings as a reliable guide in moral conflict. Under scrutiny, the Golden

Rule is not quite what it is advertised to be. First, although "Do unto others . . ." is serviceable enough in the early stages of a child's socialization, and even a moderately good rule of thumb for common daily social interactions, its application is nothing like as general as is assumed. Consider one huge domain of human action, namely defensive war. Soldiers do kill their enemies while earnestly desiring that their enemies *not* kill them. And this is regarded as the right thing for a soldier to do, though it contravenes the Golden Rule. Unfortunately, if a soldier does unto his enemies as he would be done by, he stands to be done in.

More generally, in policing and maintaining the peace, "Do unto others" applies only problematically, and usually not literally. As a police officer, I might put a child kidnapper in a headlock without at all wishing that he put me in a headlock. Likewise, jurors might feel obliged to send the accused to prison without wanting themselves to be sent to prison, even had they been similarly guilty, and so on and on.

Well, one might respond, the Golden Rule is obviously not meant to apply to *those* situations. Fine, but its claim to be universally applicable is therefore compromised, and in any case, the exception-to-the-rule problem arises again: if there are rules "all the way down," what more basic rule do we invoke in saying the Golden Rule does not apply? To what are we appealing when we claim a fairly obvious and morally acceptable exception? Perhaps, a deeper, more Golden Ur-Rule—the Platinum Rule? What would that be? As remarked earlier, knowing what is "obvious" here depends, exactly as Aristotle thought, on background common sense or moral judgment. That, however, is not a capacity that consults a set of rules to tell us when an exception is an allowable exception to the Golden Rule. Most people recognize an obvious exception when given a case, but there is no evidence that they achieve this recognition by application of a deeper rule.

There is another vast domain where the application of the Golden Rule is confusing and ambiguous at best—business and trade. While the importance of fairness in trade has long been recognized, this is largely because a good reputation is good business. As the nontrivial phrase "Business is business" implies, however, part of business is also profit, *caveat emptor*, and not being so soft-hearted that one cannot fire an employee, collect debts, or refuse credit. Running a successful business requires common sense, and common sense requires that one not literally and unconditionally apply "Do unto others" under all circumstances. Judgment and common sense are essential.

Apart from these frankly large-scale domains of activity, it is not difficult to consider many other domains where appealing to the Golden Rule is unhelpful. For example, sometimes the needs of one's own family conflict with helping others. Even if offering to take in orphans might conform to the Golden Rule, suppose that it would compromise severely the welfare of my own offspring. Do I still have a duty to take in the orphans, even if I would like to have been taken in, had I been an orphan? Does the Golden Rule tell me how to adjudicate between these options? No, not without a lot of moral filling-in that reaches deep into the Aristotelian backfill behind sensible applications of the Golden Rule.

Here is another test case: were I to need a kidney, I would surely want someone to donate her kidney to me. Does that mean I ought to donate one kidney to a stranger? A literal application of the Golden Rule says *yes*, but many virtuous people do not believe they are obliged to do this. Assorted factors go into deciding to donate a kidney, and while the Golden Rule might motivate us to consider the action, it does not settle the matter.

Were the medical staff at the Memorial Hospital in New Orleans during their terrible ordeal of hurricane Katrina applying the Golden Rule in their agonizing triage decisions?[17] It appears that they tried to do the best for the most, but with inadequate resources and little evacuation, difficult moral decisions had to be made. Some patients had to be at the bottom of the list for evacuation—not something I would want done to me, of course, but perhaps something that is least dreadful nonetheless. These sorts of cases, easily multiplied, are not silly exceptions, but significant exceptions, and they suggest that the moral understanding that underlies specific rules is more like a skill than like a concrete proposition such as "Do unto others as you would have them do unto you."

Although it is widely claimed that essentially all societies espouse the Golden Rule, this too turns out to be misleading . As philosopher Stephen Anderson notes,[18] there are negative versions and positive versions. In the negative rendition, we are asked *not* to do harm; for example in the *Analects*, what Confucius actually says is "Do not do unto others what you do not want them to do to you." This version requires much less interference and intervention by us than the positive version, such as that of Jainism, "A man should wander about treating all creatures as he himself would be treated." The positive version is a more proactive, "do-gooder" rule, and hence can be rather alarming. It enjoins us not only to avoid harming but actually to go out of our way to donate kidneys and take in orphans, while the "all creatures" clause perhaps entails that we cannot kill rats in the kitchen. Which raises the matter of exactly who "others" are, and whether they include all in my community, or all humans, or all mammals, or what. Opinions on this question vary, and the Golden Rule itself cannot settle these differences of opinion.

The deeper problem, especially with the more common positive version, concerns the variability in the moral enthusiasms humans may come to have. Here, then, is the classical flaw in the Golden Rule: there are things I would not want done to me, even by a well-meaning and dedicated follower of the positive version of the Golden Rule. That is, you might want to do something to me that *you* would indeed want done to you, but it might be something I firmly want *not* to have done to *me*—to be converted to Scientology, for example. Or to engage in sadomasochistic rituals, or be forced to be a teetotaler, or be prevented from using contraception or from choosing suicide as an end to an excruciatingly painful terminal illness, or, in the early nineteenth century, to be prevented from getting a smallpox vaccination or having anesthesia during a Caesarian section lest I end up in hell.[19] In the early part of the twentieth century, well-meaning Canadian bureaucrats removed Indian children from their homes and families and put them in residential schools in cities such as Winnipeg and Edmonton, in expectation of integrating them into the wider white society. They thought that was what they themselves would have wanted, had they been living in camps in the bush. The results were unequivocally catastrophic. A do-gooder dedicated to some crackpot ideology may feel that "were she me, she should indeed" be gassed to death or sent to live in a gulag, or given tea laced with strychnine, and proceed to arrange that fate for me. We saw quite a lot of that in the last century. The dedicated ideologue's views of what is good for me, and what he would want for himself if in my shoes, do not necessarily coincide with my own considered views.

What these last examples demonstrate is that when we extol the Golden Rule, we assume that both sides are decent, not twisted; that both sides have much the same set of moral values; that others feel about things as we do. This assumption, note, is *not* morally neutral, but contains moral content—content independent of the Golden Rule itself. Moreover, it is a sad fact of life that this assumption of universal decency does not always hold, or at least does not always look the same, even among those who advertise themselves as morally upstanding. Unfortunately, there is no shortage of ideological extremists and religious cultists and sadomasochists and sociopaths, and they can apply the Golden Rule as rigorously as anyone else.

None of these worries entails that *as a rule of thumb,* "Do unto others" is useless. To encourage a child to take the other's perspective, we say, "How would you feel if Sally did that to you?" One explanation for some version of the Golden Rule appearing in many societies is that in social life, taking into account how others will feel and respond to something we do is crucially important, as we saw in chapter 6. Predicting how others will react is prudentially wise because a reputation for being kind, fair, and hard-working versus being mean-spirited, a cheater, and a shirker, for example, has a major impact on whether one prospers or not.[20] Making it a habit to be sensitive to other's needs and feelings, a habit we try to instill in children, is also morally wise.

So the basic answer concerning why moral philosophers have not simply accepted the Golden Rule as the unconditional, universally applicable rule to guide what we ought to do is quite simple: it is *not* unconditionally and universally applicable. In many cases, such as the Memorial Hospital tragedy, the Golden Rule just does not get us very far. Worse, in cases where the do-gooder is a besotted ideologue, his application of the Golden Rule may give him precisely the justification he wants for doing what others regard as absolutely heinous things, such as engaging in genocide with the best will in the world.

Kant and His Categorical Imperative

Immanuel Kant's (1724–1804) celebrated *categorical imperative* aims to specify a completely exceptionless, unconditional (hence *categorical*) rule for moral behavior. Like others before him, most notably David Hume,[21] Kant recognized that fairness is important in morality. Hume's point was that we cannot argue that something is right for me and wrong for you just because "I am me and you are you." There has to be, at the very least, a morally relevant difference between us. For example, it is not considered fair to say "Others should pay taxes, but not me because I am *me*." Kant recognized the importance of evenhandedness in moral duty, but what was special about his approach was that he thought he saw a way to leverage evenhandedness into a grand moral theory.

Kant's conviction was that the faculty of pure reason, completely detached from any emotion or moral feeling, can use the abstract idea of the universal applicability of moral rules to establish a criterion for selecting which substantive rules define our real moral duties. Thus his categorical imperative (meaning, "what everyone ought to do, no exceptions") is actually a kind of filter that is supposed to separate the moral from the immoral rules.[22] How does pure reason achieve this result? The candidate rules that pass through Kant's proposed "filter" are all and only those rules that can be *consistently* "will" to be faithfully adopted by everyone in the moral community. Kant's emphasis on consistency here adverts to the rationality of looking out for your own well-being. His idea is that you cannot consistently affirm a rule if its observance would undermine your own well-being. Resolving to live by such a rule would be irrational. Miraculously, in Kant's scheme, precisely the set of consistent, universally binding rules *are* the moral rules.

This would indeed be a miraculous result, but as with most touted miracles, the promise turns out to be vastly greater than the product delivered. A clear test of the idea that the consistently universalizable rules are the moral rules is this: can we characterize a universally binding rule that is an obviously *im*moral rule (i.e., for present purposes, you and I agree it is immoral) and yet is a rule someone could adopt without contradiction or irrationality? As has long been known, the answer is *yes*.

Let us approach this in steps. Consider the possible rule that "All anencephalic neonates with painful terminal cancer should be euthanized." A Kantian might assume that my faculty of reason could not espouse such a rule, because were I an anencephalic neonate with painful terminal cancer, I would be ruling in favor of my own death (purportedly, an inconsistency and hence an irrationality). But in fact, I may rationally believe that were I an anencephalic neonate with painful terminal cancer, I should indeed be euthanized. Not even a faint odor of logical inconsistency or irrationality is detectable.

Since the anencephalic rule gets through Kant's filter, we have now a recipe for constructing a whole lot of other rules—some, alas, exceptionally nasty—that will pass through too. Here is the recipe: agree that the rule applies to oneself, even if it means death. This is really just the simple recognition that many people believe that there are things worse than death—dishonor, going to hell, being in terrible pain, and so forth. So merely substitute for "anencephalic neonate" a description such as "Tutsi" or "infidel" and you see that the Kantian filter cannot but let through a lot of consistent fascists as well as legions of rationally consistent moral zealots.[23]

These problems suggest that counting on pure rationality and consistency to undergird morality is mistaken.[24] In any case, Kant's conviction that detachment from emotions is essential in characterizing moral obligation is strikingly at odds with what we know about our biological nature. As we noted earlier, from a biological point of view, basic emotions are Mother Nature's way of orienting us to do what we prudentially ought. The *social* emotions are a way of getting us to do what we *socially* ought, and the reward/punishment system is a way of learning to use past experiences to improve our performance in both domains.

Consequentialism and Maximizing Utility

Jeremy Bentham (1748–1832) proposed an unconditional rule that says, in its simplest version, that one ought to act so as to produce the greatest happiness for the greatest number. This statement is what many people understand by utilitarianism, where *utility* in this context refers roughly to happiness or well-being. *Consequentialism* is the general name given to the view that it is the consequences of an action that are morally relevant, as opposed to conformity to a sacred text, for example.

In Bentham's formulation, and in that of some contemporary consequentialists, *maximizing* utility is what we are obliged to aim for in our choices generally. Although John Stuart Mill (1806–73) is most famously associated with utilitarianism, Mill scholarship shows that Mill's insight into social life was profound, and that he departed quite radically from Bentham's maximizing rule.[25] What Mill actually affirmed as the principle of utility was that the only thing that is desirable *as an end in itself* is happiness. Incidentally, it is a view that echoes Aristotle's much earlier claim that the *summum bonum* (highest good) is *eudaimonia* (roughly translatable as happiness, in the ancient sense of living well or flourishing).[26]

Two interconnected ideas account for Mill's explicit rejection of maximizing requirements for decisions in general.[27] First, for Mill, the moral sphere is fundamentally about conduct that injures, damages, or harms others or their interests. Injurious conduct, such as assault and murder, is wrong and is punishable. Conduct that falls outside this domain should be neither restricted nor deemed wrong. So on Mill's view I ought not poison my neighbor's water supply, for that would obviously damage him. On the other hand, I am not obliged to forgo playing the guitar, since this action (normally, anyhow) is not harmful to others, even though some substitute action might produce more aggregate happiness. A *maximizing* consequentialist might say my playing the guitar *is* harmful in the grotesquely extended sense that I could achieve greater aggregate happiness by forgoing my practice and working in a soup kitchen or a TB clinic. For Mill, however, this is an absurd extension of what we mean by "harmful conduct," and I do nothing wrong if I choose to go about my musical practice. Unless of course my neighbor is pinned under his tractor and desperately needs my help to survive, whereupon I will seek help. Normally, however, such needs are rare, and heeding emergencies is quite different from the unremitting maximizing that adherence to Bentham's rules implies. Judgment, as Aristotle counseled, is essential, since what counts as an emergency or an exception is not specified by a rule, but learned by examples.

Secondly, for Mill, issues of self-defense—and hence morality—are tightly tied to issues concerning acceptable restrictions on personal liberty.[28] In Mill's considered opinion, the sole end for which liberty may be restricted is self-defense, that is, defense against harmful, damaging, or injurious behavior. I may, therefore, be prevented from poisoning my neighbor's well, but not from firing a chronically and irredeemably shiftless employee. Firing him may cause harm to the employee, but preventing me from doing it on grounds that it would harm the lazy employee and his interests would be an infringement of my liberty as a business owner. Mill's account of wrongdoing does not prohibit such an action, nor does his account prohibit conduct that merely annoys others, such as competition in the marketplace or lobbying to have the Pope arrested for being an accessory to crimes.[29]

The point of emphasis then is that Mill's approach does not label an action as wrong on grounds that some other possible action might produce greater aggregate happiness. Mill's integration of his ideas concerning liberty with his ideas about moral wrongdoing make us realize how very problematic is a rule for maximizing aggregate happiness.[30] So far as advocating an absolute *rule* is concerned, therefore, Mill turns out to be less like Bentham than he is like Aristotle, identifying wrongdoing in discussion of prototypical examples rather than by rules.

Though regularly claiming Mill as an intellectual father, maximizing consequentialists run afoul of his deeper understanding of the compounded complexities of social life, and in particular of his abiding conviction concerning the social importance of liberty. Of course they may not *like* his views on liberty, but that is a different issue to be argued for on different grounds.

An enduring appeal of Mill's utilitarianism is that it acknowledges the particular importance of human *happiness*, as opposed to duty for the sake of some metaphysical end, such as pleasing God or cleansing oneself of innate sinfulness or coming back in the next life as an eagle. Philosopher Donald Brown amplifies the point: "one main thrust of this theory is to exclude from moral consideration much of what needs to be excluded: blasphemy, family honour, realpolitik, obscenity, and fictitious entities."[31] In a very broad way, much about consequentialism, absent foolishness about maximizing aggregate happiness, seems entirely ordinary and sensible. After all, we generally take it to be a benchmark of someone's rationality that he evaluates the consequences of a plan; by and large, human well-being or happiness counts for a lot in most of our socially significant decisions, and like Mill, we feel obliged to go very carefully if an action could have damaging consequences for others. *Maximizing* consequentialism in the Bentham fashion, however, takes us well beyond what is ordinary and sensible. To see this, it may be useful to look a little more closely at its rendering of our obligations in terms of maximizing aggregate happiness.

First is the practical drawback. Performing the required calculation in a way serious enough actually to qualify as maximizing happiness is a nightmare. For example, no one has the slightest idea how to compare the mild headaches of five million against the broken legs of three, or the needs of one's own two children against the needs of a hundred unrelated brain-damaged children in Serbia. And one might question: are these sorts of "far afield" calculations really necessary, *always*, in the practice of moral decency as we navigate our way through the social world? Did Socrates or Confucius, both examples of morally good humans, calculate as maximizing consequentialists decree? And am I obliged to give up one kidney for an unknown person who will otherwise die? Or even for a known person who would otherwise die? Must I convert most of my house to a shelter for derelict soldiers? Is it okay if I make a charitable donation to my local school, or must it be to a more needy clinic in Uganda? This raises the problems connected with treating all affected by my choice as having an equal claim.

Many maximizing consequentialists, such as philosopher Peter Singer,[32] argue that maximizing happiness of *all* requires that we do much more than consider the consequences of a plan for the happiness of those near and dear. According to him, in calculating consequences, everyone—*everyone*—with an interest in the consequences should be treated equally. Awkwardly, this implies that I must not put the well-being of my children ahead of that of unknown strangers living on the other side of the planet. Singer does realize that parents and children have a special relationship, but he sees that as consistent with his view, since, he argues, better consequences ensue if parents take care of their children before taking care of others. Even so, according to Singer's principles, it seems that I am obliged *not* to send my child to a private college if I could send him and two Thai children to a state college, and I am obliged *not* to get orthodontic treatment for my child if I could get basic dental care for five Haitian children. Even if I give to charity, Singer would urge that I could, surely, always give more by doing without those luxuries of life such as a new computer or a vacation. And so forth.

Singer's maximizing consequentialism is *much* more demanding, and much more meddlesome, than the morally moderate, such as I, find reasonable. The urgings of the ardent utilitarians sometimes alarm me the way intrusive do-gooders can be alarming, not least because of infringements on liberty and the conflict with paradigmatically good sense. Admittedly, however, it is not always clear to me what exactly Singer, or maximizing consequentialism in general, does require.[33] What *is* clear is that the idea of equal consideration for all goes very deep in many versions of consequentialism. As Thomas Scanlon says, the thesis is that *"all that counts morally* is the well-being of individuals, no one of whom is singled out as counting for more than the others."[34]

Finally, depending on background conditions, the maximizing consequentialist rule can run afoul of other cherished themes, such as "Punish only the guilty," or "Respect privacy," or "Harvest organs from the dead only if they or their family have given consent" or "Never change the deceased's will even if its provisions are wasteful and the wealth could be put to better use," as it asks me to maximize everyone's well-being given a particular dilemma. Some contemporary maximizers say "Fine, the Greatest Happiness rule *should* trump all other rules and moral themes"; others are less comfortable with certain possible applications. Hence there are constant fierce debates on these issues. Many moral philosophers have tried to modify aspects of the theory to make it precise, workable, understandable, and universally applicable. Brilliant though some of these maximizing attempts are, none has entirely succeeded, partly because they cannot seem to avoid requiring us to do things that a morally decent person would not do. On the other hand, the ill that comes from adopting Mill's more moderate approach may be vastly less than the ill of conforming to a rule, such as "Obey God."

In my view, consequentialism is most useful if it is espoused not as an exceptionless *rule*, but as a cluster of exemplary *moral prototypes*, cases where we can agree that calculating the prototypically good consequences (those concerning well-being) serves us well. Then, as with nonmoral categories, from the prototypes we can extend to new cases by analogy, sensitive to multiple constraints. Of course there are bound to be disagreements as we approach the fuzzy boundaries of a category. Thus someone may try to claim a harm as a result of his neighbor's working on the Sabbath, but these sorts of boundary cases are *not* best resolved by trying to maximize aggregate utility.[35] Nevertheless, as Mill rightly saw, pointing out the consequences for human well-being, however difficult to quantify precisely, is always pertinent.

What worried Mill, and worries me, are the moral claims, often espoused stoutly and dogmatically, that fly in the face of human well-being. As a child, I found the prototype of perversity to be the rule that you must do what God commands. Particularly worrisome was its application in the Bible story of Abraham and Isaac, a story served up in Sunday school to my six-year-old ears. Abraham thinks he hears God command him to take his beloved son Isaac into the hills and slay him with a knife and burn him as a sacrifice. Heeding the call, he takes Isaac into the hills. In the nick of time, an angel luckily announces that God wants him to spare Isaac's life after all. To the child's mind, it seemed obvious that the God in question was terrifying and untrustworthy, and that Abraham was a deranged nitwit. I was relieved that my father showed no sign of communicating with God or angels and was otherwise disinclined to theological enthusiasms. Later, I found other grim lessons in ideological fervor that disregarded human well-being while proclaiming otherwise. Such, for example, were the horrors visited upon Chinese scientists and intellectuals, not to mention many others, during the Cultural Revolution in China launched by Mao Zedong in 1966.

History, and even current societies, provide no end of examples of rules requiring things that appear to be contrary to the well-being of citizens. Surprisingly often, well-being is not terribly hard to assess.[36] Killing female rape victims, for example, does not serve anyone's well-being, nor does prohibiting measles and polio vaccinations or the use of condoms. Allowing military assault weapons to be purchased by ordinary citizens does not serve anyone's well-being. Installing early warning devices for a tsunami does serve the well-being of many. Allowing genes to be patented probably does not serve the well-being of humans in the long run, but that is less clear-cut. In many other cases, well-being can be difficult to settle, especially when a practice is deeply entrenched in an institution with a long and esteemed history, making it difficult to get agreement on what serves human well-being in the long run.

Again, philosopher Owen Flanagan is wise on this matter. When there is conflict about what option best serves human well-being, he asks, where does one go for clarification? To the guru on the mountaintop, a favorite of cartoonists? To an alleged holy man? Flanagan's answer is, "to the world. There is no other place to go."[37] What does he mean by that? His point is that the process of reflecting on alternatives, understanding history and humans needs, seeing things from the perspective of others, and talking it through with others can lead us to better evaluations of a social practice in the long run. Better, that is, than relying on self-appointed moral authorities and their list of rules. This process can sometimes change our minds, and even the institutions that venerate the practice.[38] What does not exist is a Platonic Heaven wherein the Moral Truths reside—no more than that there is a Platonic Heaven wherein the Physical Truths reside.

Facts about Rule Use

Do normal, sensible, competent people decide what they ought to do without appeal to rules? Yes indeed. Not just occasionally, not just under bizarre conditions, but regularly and effectively, in both prudential and moral domains.[39] For a prudential example, when I see red pebbly spots on my child's leg, I immediately realize that I ought to apply an antihistamine ointment because I recognize the rash to be a reaction to contact with poison ivy. The decision relies in part on memory of earlier instances that are relevantly similar to this one, and knowledge of the local flora. The case-based memory, whether conscious or not, is tagged with the negative valuation of a case of poison ivy allowed to run unchecked. The decision is context sensitive. That is, if more urgent events suddenly occur, such as the appearance of a rabid dog at the door or a fire on the stove, then applying antihistamine gets lower priority than shooting the rabid dog at the door or dousing a house fire. Case-based reasoning involves drawing on a remembered prototype that resembles the case at hand, and filling in the similarity with a similar response.[40] Moreover, the brain often relies on case-based reasoning when we cannot articulate exactly what the facts are. For example, a friend's father makes an odd comment to me, and something about his demeanor and comment triggers a faint memory and a small alarm. I think I ought to give this man a wide berth, and not get too friendly. I cannot say precisely why. I am just being prudent. What rule am I appealing to? None that I know of.

While exceptionless rules are frequently considered necessary in the moral domain, nobody appears to suppose they are needed for *prudential*, everyday, nonmoral, *oughts*. We manage our interactions with the physical world quit well without ground-floor, exceptionless rules. Roughly speaking, broody hens ought to be removed from the flock, yeast ought to be kept in the refrigerator, tire pressure ought to be checked every month, teeth ought to be flossed after meals, skunks ought to be given a wide berth, tetanus shots should be updated every seven years, and so on and bloody on. So if we can determine what prudentially we ought to do, without aid of an exceptionless prudential rule, why not in the moral domain?[41]

Here is a mundane *moral* "ought," determined from a set of facts, using ordinary case-based reasoning. My neighbor is away, and I see the deer have breached the fence and are browsing on his young apple trees. I know he does not want his orchard destroyed by deer, so I interrupt my work, call my dogs, grab a broom, chase out the deer, and make a temporary mend on the fence. I decide what I ought to do without consulting a foundational rule, such as "Always chase deer out of orchards" or "Always help the neighbors."

A strategy for probing how people make moral decisions consists in contriving moral dilemmas designed to pit *kill-one-to-save-many* against *kill-no-one-and-let-many-die*. Subjects read the scenarios and then rate the moral propriety of the alternatives. Not surprisingly, responses vary. The dominant interpretation of the main variation is that some (those who refuse to kill one to save many) have an automatic and emotional adherence to rules while others (those who would kill one to save many) employ reason to decide, and are less governed by rules or emotions. The scenarios are stripped of any details about the individuals, their history, the context, the law of the land, the ramifications on reputation, etc. The detail-stripping is intended to eliminate confounds, but it introduces a new flaw: the scenario is so artificial that the brain's normal reliance on morally relevant facts to guide problem-solving is undermined.

A more plausible interpretation is this: everyone uses case-based reasoning, but given our individual histories and temperaments, we may draw on different cases to guide judgment concerning the present case. One student may respond negatively to "sacrifice one for many," having learned about needless sacrifices made by Russians during the Communist era. Another student may respond positively based on an association with a movie of a torpedoed submarine in which all would drown unless the engine room door were sealed, dooming the engineer. Other prototypes might edge their way into the minds of individual subjects, tilting them a little one way or another. Rules may be invoked after the fact but only to satisfy a social expectation of a rule-based explanation. If, as I suspect, the moral dilemmas we encounter in the real world are typically resolved by constraint-satisfaction, then case-based analogies, emotions, memory, and imagination are almost always involved.[42]

An illustration of my point about the role of rules emerged, without warning and to much amusement, in an interview of Georgia representative Lynn Westmoreland on the TV satiric show *The Colbert Report*. The topic of Stephen Colbert's extended discussion with Westmoreland was a recent higher-court ban on the public display of the Ten Commandments in the foyer of a Louisiana courthouse, and the justice or injustice of their subsequent court-ordered removal. The congressman was defending their public, cast-bronze-on-granite display on a variety of grounds, but most trenchantly on the grounds that, collectively, those ten rules constitute the very foundation of our morality, insofar as we have any morality. Their public display, therefore, could only serve to enhance the level of individual morality.

Sensing an opportunity, Stephen Colbert nodded his presumptive assent to this claim, and asked his guest, "Could you please cite them for us, Congressman?" Westmoreland, plainly taken aback by the request, gamely began ". . . Don't lie, . . . don't steal, . . . don't kill, . . . ," as Colbert, with his eyebrows raised in expectation, held up first one finger in response, then two, then three. After an awkward pause at that point, the congressman, who had plainly drawn a blank beyond those three, bravely and with evident honesty said, "No, I'm sorry. I can't name them all." At which point Colbert ostentatiously thanked his guest for his wisdom and brought the interview to an uproariously received and laughter-filled conclusion.

The irony was plain enough and doesn't need any further elaboration from me. But there is a deeper lesson to be drawn from this exchange. The fact is, the congressman is probably as good an example of worthy moral character as one is likely to encounter at one's local post office or grocery store. After all, he inspired sufficient public trust to get himself elected, and he thinks morality important enough to defend it, with some passion and resourcefulness, on television. (Note, however, that it was Westmoreland who, in an interview during the last presidential campaign, described Barack Obama as "uppity," a remark generally construed as a racial slur.) But if he is a presumptive example of a conscientious man, his welcome virtues are clearly *not* owed to his carrying around, in memory, a specific list of discursive rules, rules at his immediate command, rules that he literally consults in order to guide his ongoing social behavior. After all, he could remember only three of the ten "commandments" at issue, and, according to my copy of the Bible, he didn't get two of those quite right in any case. If we are looking for an explanation of the actual ground of people's moral behavior, the proposal that we are all following a specific set of discursive rules in order to produce that behavior looks strained and threadbare, to put it mildly.

Normativity and the Moral "Ought"

Agreeing with Robert Solomon that the very definition of morality involves rules, Bernard Gert, in his entry in the *Stanford Encyclopedia of Philosophy* under the heading "The Definition of Morality," begins his discussion:

> The term "morality" can be used either
>
> 1. *descriptively* to refer to a code of conduct put forward by a society or,
>   a. some other group, such as a religion, or
>   b. accepted by an individual for her own behavior or
> 2. *normatively* to refer to a code of conduct that, given specified conditions, would be put forward by all rational persons.[43]

The distinction between descriptions and norms—between what is and what ought to be—is accepted as obvious and unbridgeable in contemporary moral philosophy, as noted earlier in chapter 1.[44] Mainstream moral philosophers tend to regard the description of a culture's social codes as of mainly anthropological interest, and not at the heart of morality in its profound, normative sense—what rule(s) *ought* to be followed. Likewise, the descriptions of the neurobiology of sociality are considered merely as descriptions of what is, and hence can tell us nothing about what we ought to do. It is the normative project—specifying the rule(s) that would be accepted by all rational persons—that is embraced as the intellectual calling of moral philosophy, as exemplified by Peter Singer and John Rawls. This privileged focus on the normative project is largely explained by near-universal acceptance of the idea that the distinction between *is* and *ought*—between facts and values, between the descriptive and the normative—entails that the normative project is ultimately autonomous with respect to descriptions of the facts. Facts are in the world to be observed, but not so rules. No rules, then no (genuinely) moral decisions. Sensitive to the argument that morality cannot originate in divine commands, moral philosophers have instead looked to rationality as the source of adequate moral rules.

Given their convictions about the autonomy of the normative domain, many moral philosophers regard the fact/value distinction as effectively scotching the entire enterprise in this book. Wrong though I believe them to be, I take these reservations very seriously, and will analyze the arguments in the next section.

The Naturalistic Fallacy

Philosophers have long argued that naturalism in ethics—appealing to our natures to address the fundamental values—rests on a mistake, an almost stupid mistake. According to the most famous version, naturalism involves a simple fallacy, known widely and taught routinely as the *Naturalistic Fallacy*, a term coined by the British philosopher G. E. Moore.[45] The Naturalistic Fallacy consists in supposing that properties such as the good or right or valuable can be identified with some *natural* property or set of properties, such as happiness or flourishing or love; for example, Aristotle thought the most basic good was happiness (flourishing). Any attempt of this kind, according to Moore's argument, is obviously fallacious, as he supposed could readily be seen by mulling over the following point: for any statement identifying a natural property as the property of being *good*, or *valuable*, for example "Happiness is good," or "Love is valuable," there is always a perfectly reasonable open question: "But *is* happiness good?" or "Is love valuable?" If the two properties (e.g., goodness and happiness) really were identical, any competent speaker would know that, and a question such as "Is happiness good?" would be silly. But the question "Is happiness good?" is not silly. Therefore, he said, the properties could not be identical.[46] The really deep point, according to Moore, is that *there is no answer to the question of what natural properties are identical with the good or the right or the valuable*. That is because for any proposal, the open question can always be asked. Allegedly, our only recourse to what is *right* or *good* consists in referring to the brute fact of our intuitions. According to Moore, the bedrock of intuition laid bare by the open question argument means that "good" is a *non-natural property*—that is, a property that cannot be studied by science, in the way that prosperity, for example, can be studied by science. Calling moral intuitions a *brute* fact was his way of affirming that such intuitions cannot be explained. Non-natural properties can be studied by philosophers (like himself) but not by scientists.

Having created a mystical moat around moral behavior, Moore cheerfully expanded on what is fallacious in naturalism: if the property of being pleasurable were identical to the property of being good, then the meaning of "happiness" and "good" would be the same. It would be like saying that being a bachelor is the same as being an unmarried man. But if that were true, he said, then the statement "Happiness is good" would be equivalent to "Happiness is happiness," and it would be entirely uninformative. But saying happiness is good *is* informative, and is not trivial, says Moore. The fallacy, he concluded, could not be more evident. This, Moore figured, meant that any attempt to identify natural properties with what is valuable or good is wrecked on the shoals of the Naturalistic Fallacy.

Moore's theory about non-natural properties reinforced a conventionally appealing background presumption that values are completely separate from facts, and the companion idea that facts about our natures cannot tell us anything about what is truly valuable. Although Moore's arguments are flawed, as I shall discuss below, his separation of science and moral philosophy established itself as orthodoxy; one crossed that boundary only by falling for the Naturalistic Fallacy.

In the twentieth century, moral philosophy advertised itself as a *normative* discipline, concerned with what ought to be done, and especially with foundational rules of morality. Roughly, many moral philosophers believed that just as science can tell us nothing fundamental about what is good or valuable, it can tell us nothing about how we ought to live. It might tell us something about what some tribe believes is good, but it is always an *open question* whether that genuinely is good. It might tell us how to *get* what is valuable, but the value itself is beyond science. This was Moore's unfortunate legacy.

Moore's arguments, when examined closely, are strange. For example, his claim that to say that A is B requires synonymy of the terms A and B is utterly contrived. It clearly does not hold when the A and B are scientific terms. To see this, consider these scientifically demonstrated identifications: light (A) is electromagnetic radiation (B), or temperature (A) is mean molecular kinetic energy (B). Here, the A and B terms are not synonymous, but the property measured one way was found to be the same as the property measured another way. The claims are factual claims, ones in which a factual discovery is made. Consider a more everyday sort of case: Suppose I discover that my neighbor Bill Smith (A) is in fact the head of the CIA (B): are the expressions "my neighbor Bill Smith" and "the head of the CIA" synonymous? Of course not.

What would be an example where, if I say "A is the same as B," the expressions A and B must be synonymous? The best example is one in which we make a semantic, not a factual claim, e.g., if A is "the meaning of STOP" and B is "the meaning of ARRETE," and I say "The meaning of STOP is the same as the meaning of ARRETE." Poor Moore would have realized that this sort of example was no support for his point. The upshot of all this is that if identifications in general do not require synonymy of terms, whyever should they in the domain of morality? And if they do not, then the wheels fall off Moore's argument.

Needless to say, not all proposed identifications in science are true: viruses are not bacteria, and temperature is not caloric fluid. So perhaps it was the simplicity of the particular instances of identifications of *valuable* with, for example, *pleasure*, that drew Moore into a wholly muddled theory about identifications and his odd ideas about "non-natural properties." Our brains, and the brains of animals generally, are organized to value survival and well-being; survival and well-being are valuable. Our perceptions are permeated with value, and in that sense they are valenced.[47]

Had Moore merely pointed out that the relation between our nature and what is good is complex, not simple, he would have been on firmer ground. Analogously, the relation between our nature and health is complex. As with morals and values, no simple formula will suffice. Because one cannot simply equate health with, for example, low blood pressure or getting enough sleep, a Moore-on-health might argue that *health* is a non-natural property—unanalyzable and metaphysically autonomous. Using science to help figure out what we *ought* to do to be healthy will, on this Moorean view, be unrewarding, since that is an "ought" project—a normative, not a factual project. Such a view seems peculiar, of course, and it is so even though there are many aspects of healthy living where disagreement persists, such as the degree to which play or meditation contribute to mental health, whether alcoholism should be considered a disease, whether statins should be prescribed for everyone over fifty, how placebos work, how thin is too thin, and so forth. Disagreements notwithstanding, we know quite a lot about what we ought to do to be healthy, based on facts made available by science.

As the biological sciences have advanced, we have come to know more about health, and about what kinds of conditions contribute to staving off or curing certain diseases. As knowledge about individual differences, and about the relation between features in the environment and particular medical conditions, begin to emerge, we start to appreciate just how very complex the topic of human health really is. It is a domain where science can teach us, and has already taught us, a great deal about what we ought to do.

Likewise, the domain of social behavior is very complex, and we may learn a great deal from common observation and from science about conditions favoring social harmony and stability, and about individual quality of life. Nothing in Moore's argument shows otherwise. Indeed, from the perspective of evolutionary biology, Moore's retreat to unanalyzable intuition as the basis for morality looks unpromising, to put it politely. Intuitions, after all, are products of the brain—they are not miraculous channels to the Truth. They are generated in some way by nervous systems; they are undoubtedly dependent on experience and cultural practices, however hidden from consciousness the causes may be. That we cannot introspect their source is just a fact about brain function—about what is and is not conscious. It implies nothing concerning the Metaphysical Truth about what those intuitions tell us.

None of this discussion implies that science can solve all moral dilemmas, nor even that scientists or philosophers are morally wiser than farmers or carpenters. But it does suggest that we should be open to the possibility that a deeper understanding of the nature of our sociality may shed light on certain of our practices and institutions, and cause us to think more wisely about them.

8. Religion and Morality

Morality seems to me to be a natural phenomenon—constrained by the forces of natural selection, rooted in neurobiology, shaped by the local ecology, and modified by cultural developments. Nevertheless, fairness requires me to acknowledge that this sort of naturalistic approach to morality has often seemed insensitive to metaphysical ideas about morality, such as that morality is essentially dependent on a supernatural source of moral information and moral worth. Because this is a not uncommon view, it may be useful to consider what a supernatural approach can teach us.

Conscience and Morality

When asked, most humans can easily tell a story of a morally decent or morally courageous act. Stories may come from our own lives, where a neighbor intervened to rescue a lad from brutal beatings by a drunken father or the village pooled its meager resources to build a school and hire a teacher. Or we may retell an oft-told tale, of Schindler shielding Jews from the Gestapo, of Atticus Finch defending Tom Robinson against the charge of raping a white woman in Harper Lee's novel, *To Kill A Mockingbird*, of Horatio standing doomed but courageous at the bridge, of Dr. Ignaz Semmelweis's (1840s) attempts to convince his hostile colleagues that hand-washing before examining maternity patients reduced death from childbed fever. Frequently, we have no trouble recognizing the difference between admirable thrift and craven stinginess, or between fair-minded leadership and self-aggrandizing displays of power. Lines can get fuzzy, however, for just about any category, moral or otherwise. We ask: is this plan appeasement or diplomacy? Is this fibbing or common courtesy?

Conscience, it is sometimes believed, is our guide in moral decisions. So far, so good. A further and additional claim, however, may be that morality *originates* in the human conscience, and as a gift from God, conscience is an entity that encapsulates the natural law that God wishes us to follow.[1] Conscience, a God-given entity, throws its weight for or against a plan; it keeps us from succumbing to temptation. Conscience, we are sometimes advised, will always guide us aright, if only we listen to what it is *really* saying. That, the story goes, is because we are all given the same moral conscience as a birthright. Thus there are usually two parts to this conscience thesis: (1) that we often have strong feelings about what is right and wrong, and (2) that there is a sort of metaphysical entity, conscience, that can be counted on for morally correct solutions to moral dilemmas.

The first part of the "conscience" account is entirely in keeping with what we know about social learning in normal humans. As argued in earlier chapters, given normal neural networks, the pain from being shunned and the pleasure of belonging, along with imitation of those we admire, give rise to powerful intuitions about the absolute rightness or wrongness of classes of behavior. This scheme of responses, much of which takes form during brain-gene-environment interactions as the child begins to live its social life, is the neurobiological reality behind our talk of *conscience*. Unhitched from the neurobiology of sociality and social learning, however, conscience, as a *metaphysical* entity with moral knowledge, loses its footing.

One long-standing difficulty with this idea, as Socrates (469–399 BCE) ruefully acknowledged, is that our *inner voices* do not always advise the same way—not the same as other individuals, or even the same as ourselves over time—even when we *really* listen to them. Inner voices are sensitive to community standards, and those vary between and within cultures. One person's inner voice tells him that when willing noncombatants act as shields for combatants, soldiers may treat them as combatants; another's inner voice sees such a policy as undermining the legitimacy of the soldiers' role in the conflict. One person's inner voice makes no objection to eating domestic fowl; another person's inner voice is horrified at meat-eating. According to legend, playwright George Bernard Shaw's conscience spoke to him, "animals are my friends, and I do not eat my friends." On the other hand, growing up on a poor farm where meat was a luxury, I quickly learned to wring the necks of the hens I daily and lovingly fed.[2] My inner voice and Shaw's gave different directives. Some inner voices seem to have more compassion than others. Some display a live-and-let-live profile. Others demand strict and inflexible adherence to rules. Sometimes conscience does not guide, and the conflict between choices remains painfully unresolved: should the underling blow the whistle on corruption and jeopardize a career and perhaps a life?

The inner voice of conscience is sensitive to advances in knowledge and to maturing experiences. It is sensitive to drugs and sleep deprivation. The inner voice seems to be more like auditory imagination, aided by visual imagination of the consequences of a choice, generated by the brain as it exercises its problem-solving capacity, rather than like the pure pronouncements of a brain-independent, metaphysically separate Platonic storehouse of moral knowledge. In the next section, I consider whether the metaphysical approach might be more successful if it shifts weight to the metaphysics of a supernatural deity.

Morality and Religion

A related and perhaps more widespread view is that religion is the source of the moral principles for our lives; rightness and wrongness are what they are only because of a Divine Being.

According to the doctrinal beliefs of some religions, morality is imposed by God on wicked and unwilling humans for their own good, with threat of punishment for the noncompliant. In certain versions of this doctrine, the rules supplied by the deity are tangential to human happiness in the earthly domain. As the preacher Franklin (son of Billy) Graham has said, it is far better to please God, rather than ourselves, no matter the cost.[3] Thus in some doctrines, the moral principles specify a way of life needed for access to an afterlife, but are indifferent to suffering here and now. Cultural differences in certain principles are, accordingly, sometimes explained—on both sides of a cultural divide—as errors, such as having linked up with the wrong sort of god, or not the real God, or as having misunderstood what God intended. This has not always made for cordiality.

Religions in which a metaphysics of divine beings has a minor place typically have a more worldly view of the origins of morality and the point of morality. Exemplary human figures such as Buddha or Confucius are admired as exceptionally wise persons, not gods. They can be counted on for useful and sound advice, though not for hidebound rules, about how to live a virtuous life. In these metaphysics-light religions, moral wisdom is human, but hard won and full of complexity. Depending on the sect, living the good life may be important for events in the hereafter, but most likely it is important mainly for making the best of life here and now, and perhaps especially important for the well-being of future generations.

In metaphysics-heavy traditions, the connection between God and morality has sometimes been regarded as axiomatic. Socrates, always questioning the allegedly obvious, suspected it was anything but. He was moved to ponder the exact role of the gods in morality, and his worried discussion was captured by Plato in his magnificent dialogue, *The Euthyphro*.

Envision the scene: Socrates is strolling to court, to face charges of corrupting the youth of Athens. In fact, however, he has merely embarrassed some self-important authorities by questioning the "conventional wisdom." Socrates, ever realistic, accurately predicts his conviction on the charges, and finally, his execution by poison. Facing the legal punishment of death is the most poignant occasion to inquire into the fundamentals of ethics: What is justice? Where do moral laws come from? What is the root of moral motivation? What is the relation between power and morality?

As he goes to court, Socrates is joined by Euthyphro, a clever and self-satisfied priest. The setting is particularly apt for a discussion of morality, and not only because of Socrates' impending conviction. Euthyphro, it turns out, is going to court to prosecute his own father for having thrown a slave in a ditch. The case is full of moral ambiguity — a loving father stands to be publicly rebuked by an arrogant son, where the matter of abuse of a slave might have been better resolved gently and within the family. Socrates is as mystified by the unwavering moral pompousness of Euthyphro as by that of his own prosecutors. And so begins the dialogue.

To Socrates' seemingly simple question, "So, Euthyphro, tell us, what is good?"[4] Euthyphro confidently delivers the favored religious answer: the good is what the gods say is good. (Updated for monotheists, what is good is what God says is good.) Socrates presses further, however, having discerned a fatal ambiguity. He skillfully draws out the problem in the religious answer by posing his troublesome dilemma: is something good because the gods *say* that it is good (saying makes it so), or do the gods say something is good because it *is* good (they act as authoritative messengers of an independent fact)?

No fool, Euthyphro instantly recognizes the first as an untenable option, and backs away. If something's being right consists merely in the gods' *pronouncing* it right, then *any* pronouncement of the gods, however horrible from the human standpoint, is ipso facto right (e.g., suppose Zeus says, "Boil your first born baby and feed it to the dogs"). What then, of the second—the gods say something is right because in fact it *is* right? This seems more promising. Socrates pushes on, pointing out its unwelcome implications: then the *source* or origin of goodness (justice) cannot be the gods at all. The gods merely communicate, and, for all we can be sure, poorly. The trouble is, this option sheds no light on what it is about certain acts or institutions that makes them good or just. It does not help us with our moral judgment. And, even more troubling, it sheds no light on the connection between human life and morality. So why bring in the gods at all?

Always modest, Socrates confesses ignorance of the answer to his own questions concerning the source of morality. The pattern of questioning strongly hints, however, that whatever it is that makes something good or just or right is rooted in the nature of humans and the society we make, not in the nature of the gods we invent. There is something about the facts concerning human needs and human nature that entails that some social practices are better than others, that some human behavior cannot be tolerated, and that some forms of punishment are needed.[5] This does not mean that moral practices are mere conventions, on par with using a fork or wearing a hat to a funeral. Moral practices are typically pertinent in more serious situations, such as the conduct of war and the distribution of scarce resources.

A further problem with the second option (the gods as communicators) I call *the handoff problem*. If we want to get moral advice from supernatural sources, how do we *reliably* get that information? Being supernatural, the gods are not among us as part of the natural world. Most of us are disinclined to believe that we ourselves are privy to direct and clear communication with the divine. So who is privy? There is no shortage of people who *claim*, sincerely or otherwise, that they do have a special communication channel to divine commands about what we all should do. But, and this is a crucially important question, are any of these claims believable? Some of the claimants are clearly deluded, as must be said of evangelist Jim Jones, who led his devout flock to build a commune in Guyana and eventually persuaded some nine hundred of them, children included, to consume strychnine-laced fruit drink Others, such as televangelists Jimmy Swaggart and Peter Popoff, have been unmasked as frauds, fleecing the gullible. Their attempts to prove their reliability by demonstrations of faith-healing were a hoax. So how can we determine who has reliable contact with God who can deliver to the rest of us information about how God wants us behave?

Difficulties compound because even within a religious denomination, there are apt to be disagreements on many issues concerning what God commands. Protestants do not believe that God forbids contraception; doctrinally, Roman Catholics do, though in fact contraception is widely used among Catholics. Roman Catholics think the Pope is infallible when he speaks *ex cathedra*, conveying God's views via a special relationship; Protestants, Jews, and Muslims consider this mistaken. Jehovah's Witnesses believe God forbids blood transfusions, Episcopalians are reasonably sure He does not. Leviticus 25:44–46 reassures us that slavery is fine, but few Christians of any kind now take that seriously.[6] Ephesians 5:24 is unqualified: "As the church submits to Christ, so wives should submit to their husbands in everything," something not all Christians or Jews take seriously. Or how about Luke 14:26: "If any man come to me, and hate not his father, and mother, and wife, and children, and brethren, and sisters, yea, and his own life also, he cannot be my disciple." Seems a rather strong, and not very charitable, requirement. Some evangelical preachers claim special knowledge concerning what Jesus wants us to do about gun control, the military draft, Wall Street bonuses, and AIDS. George W. Bush, when president of the United States, claimed that he communicated with God concerning certain matters of state. All those who speak to God's wishes claim reliability, which suggests, given their mutual inconsistencies, that none truly are receiving their information on the clear channel.

Moreover, even when religions agree about what God commands, adherents rarely follow the commands to the letter. The Ten

Commandments, for example, include the commandment not to kill, but in practice Christians and Jews, reasonably enough, regard killing in war, self-defense, and so forth as acceptable. Whatever the status of the commandments, they cannot be exceptionless.[7] The handoff problem, therefore, is serious. Worse, it makes for great trouble when enthusiastic members of one sect feel impelled to kill diehards of another sect who disagree on what their gods say is right.

There is one further point. As noted above, not all religions see morality as god-dependent, and some have no supernatural deities at all. Hundreds of millions of the world's humans are religious in a sense that does not involve a Creator, Law-Giver, or Divine Person. Buddhism, Confucianism, Taoism, and some other Asian religions may venerate ancestors, and venerate certain apparently wise persons, or may worship the sun and moon. Some in the West are pantheists, believing that Nature is worthy of spiritual veneration, and that from living close to Nature, we undergo moral development. Such religious approaches lack the theology of a Divine Person; their moral wisdom is typically this-worldly, not other-worldly; it is about how to get on in life.[8] As such, their accumulated wisdom is open to discussion and debate, and also to continued modification to keep current with changes in the ecological conditions and in our social understanding.

A connection between religion and morality there surely is, but it appears that the connection is mainly sociological[9] rather metaphysical. In a religious context, moral issues are often raised and discussed; moral practices are conveyed to the young, and reinforced in the mature. Religious festivals can be an occasion for group bonding around certain moral issues, such as defense against attackers, celebration of a new leader, or survival during a harsh winter and distribution of scarce resources. Religious rituals are important in reaffirming social hierarchies and in solidifying social coalitions, and some religious practices are structured to increase compassion, kindness, harmony, and love.[10] As well, rituals of affiliation can ignite contagious enthusiasm for a group's undertaking and can be helpful in solving certain kinds of social problems, such as organizing defense against attack, or, as in the Crusades or the Inquisitions, organizing the attack itself. Notice, however, that these effects, fascinating though they may be, are tangential to the question at hand: *Does morality have a supernatural basis?*

Perhaps life would be a whole lot simpler if there were a divine being who could reliably be appealed to for a straight answer on moral issues, an answer made clear to all. Perhaps then the ambiguities, different perspectives, differences in background and education, the tensions of disagreement and the agonies of decision-making, could all be laid to rest, though perhaps not even then. In any case, like the fondly desired fountain of youth or the perpetual motion machine, these are mere wishes, not reality.

Thus we have no option but to wrestle with difficult social issues, to hear the other side and to heed the differences, to negotiate as wisely as we can, to understand the history, and to try to foresee future consequences. The wisdom of elders can usefully be brought into play, and some old saws have staying power: "Don't let the best be the enemy of the good"; "Don't burn your bridges behind you." Laws and institutions can be changed, but even with the best of intentions, a law can turn out to have unintended bad consequences. Sometimes there is no uniquely right answer, no uniquely good outcome, just some roughly decent ways of avoiding a worse horror.

Does This Mean Morality Is an Illusion?

According to geneticist Francis Collins, now director of the National Institutes of Health, "God gifted humanity with the knowledge of good and evil (the moral law)," and "if the moral law is just a side effect of evolution, then there is no such thing as good and evil."[11] This tends to remind one of the odd remark that if God is dead, everything is permitted.[12] The God Collins has in mind is the God of some version of Christianity, not the gods of the Haida or the Druids or the ancient Greeks or Egyptians.

On my hypothesis regarding the neural basis of moral behavior, morality is as real as can be—it is as real as social behavior. Actual human moral behavior, in all its glory and complexity, should not be cheapened by the false dilemma: either God secures the moral law or morality is an illusion. It is a false dilemma because morality can be—and I argue, *is*—grounded in our biology, in our capacity for compassion and our ability to learn and figure things out. As a matter of actual fact, some social practices are better than others, some institutions are worse than others, and genuine assessments can be made against the standard of how well or poorly they serve human well-being.[13] Allowing women to vote has, despite dire predictions of disaster, turned out reasonably well, whereas the laws allowing private citizens to own assault weapons in the United States has had quite a lot of deleterious consequences. Abolition of slavery, though a fairly recent development, is surely, as a matter of the facts of well-being, better than slavery. That some one or other may disagree on various matters does not entail that without God, all is mere opinion. In the field of science, that some disagree that the Earth is a sphere, or that it is more than six thousand years old, does not entail that these are mere matters of opinion.

What, exactly is the moral law to which to which Collins refers? The Ten Commandments, I hazard to guess, is the starting place. Aristotle saw clearly the trap awaiting the supposition that one's own religion is the one true religion and one's own moral intuitions are planted in the conscience by one's own special God. For one thing, it makes a virtue of intolerance—those who disagree regarding a matter of morals *must* be dead wrong. For another, it spawns moral arrogance at exactly those points in social life when we need humility and reflection. That I have a special relationship with God, whereby I *know* that what others do is wrong, but what I do is right and has God's blessing, is a very dangerous assumption. People holding that view may be virtuous and kind, but all too often they are moral bullies.

The next problem with the idea that without a God morality is an illusion is that many people who are not in the least adherents of a deistic religion and who may have no theological belief at all are in fact exemplary in their moral behavior. This is also true of whole societies, such as those Asian societies that espouse Confucianism, Taoism, or Buddhism, but not a deity who is a law-giver. It was true of Aristotle and Marcus Aurelius (121–180 CE) and David Hume, morally wise humans all. It is true of Unitarians and atheists. Their morality is entirely real, and to dismiss it as illusory because they do not share a metaphysics of divine beings borders on the delusional. Such self-certainly is itself morally questionable.

Chapter 3 considered the hypothesis regarding the emergence of sociality in mammals and the circuitry in the brainstem and limbic structures that extends self-care to care for offspring, and in highly social species, to care for others such as mates, kin, affiliates, and, perhaps, strangers. Aristotle did not, needless to say, know *what* it is about our physical being that makes us social by nature. He knew nothing about genes, neurons, oxytocin, and vasopressin. But like Confucius, Aristotle saw morality not as a divine business or a magical business, but as an essentially practical business. Making good laws and building good institutions he thought of as cooperative tasks requiring intelligence and understanding and a grasp of the relevant facts. He did not for a moment suppose that morality is merely an illusion. Rather, recognizing moral problems for what they are—difficult, practical problems emerging from living a social life—denies us the easy luxury of supposing God's answers are simply written in our heartfelt intuitions.

Morality, Trust, and Cultural Niche Construction

Hume "describes a partially selfish, partially sympathetic human nature, able to take into account a point of view in common with others, and able to evolve institutions that increase its security, happiness, convenience, and pleasure."[14] Simon Blackburn's discussion of David Hume shows how much Hume grasped about morality and human nature, linking the four components of successful sociality: self-care, other-care, theory of mind, and social problem-solving. The earlier chapters of this book can be seen as providing only the details, many newly discovered, to round out Hume's considerable insight. Trust between parents and children, between mates, between partners or colleagues or business associates, is overwhelmingly important in human sociality, and we now know that trust has much to do with oxytocin and vasopressin, their receptor distributions, and the complex circuitry in the limbic structures, the brainstem, and the structures of the prefrontal cortex.

In modern human social life, trust is by no means limited to kin who have proved trustworthy. Many daily interactions, from depositing money in a bank to ordering a book online to letting a doctor set a broken bone, rest on trust. How can trust extend in these ways? The first-pass answer is that we have grown up in a culture of long-established, regulated institutions, and our trust in these institutions rests on background knowledge concerning what they can be counted upon to do.[15] More simply, we have beliefs and expectations that exist because of our culture, and these involve beliefs about the trustworthiness of particular institutions and the people within them. The motherboard of trust is still the family, with trusting extensions reaching a little or a lot to other kin and friends. Yet a kind of real trust, guarded and watchful in varying degrees, does come to be extended beyond those who are familiar.

Hume understood this aspect of social behavior as well as anyone during his time. He knew that especially as human groups expand beyond small clans or villages, the creation of stable institutions that allow us to count on certain transactions, without continual assays of trustworthiness, makes it possible for people to trust others they scarcely know, and thereby enhance their well-being. In a small clan of twenty or so people, social watchfulness can effectively curb nascent inclinations to cheat or shirk. In such circumstances, a tarnished reputation can be a significant cost to prosperity of oneself and one's family, and this is easily appreciated.[16] In larger groups, however, or cities where one may have at most a passing acquaintance with a bank teller or a policeman, trust is not so much a relation between the individuals engaged in the transaction as vested in the institution that has established itself as trustworthy. When the institution is stable, inasmuch as it is supported by laws conducive to earning trust and the enforcement of those laws, then everyone involved gains. There are many reasons not to put money under the mattress, and banks are, by and large, a safe place for one's money. Occasionally, a bank employee embezzles, but auditors eventually catch it, and in a blaze of publicity, the embezzler goes to jail. Accredited anesthesiologists are, by and large, good at their jobs, and we count on medical schools to weed out the incompetent, and on hospital oversight boards to sack accredited ones that are falling down on the job. What has been so searing in the sexual abuse of children by priests, evidently widespread, is the wrenching, disorienting violation of trust.

Hume's point concerning institutions is apt to be overlooked by those who see the centerpiece of morality as either the exceptionless rule, or duty-for-the-sake-of-duty. For Hume, both of these are pie-in-the-sky preoccupations. Hume, like his fellow Scotsman Adam Smith, realized that prosperity is important in well-being, and that prosperity can be aided or hindered by the quality of the social institutions that exist—including seemingly unglamorous institutions such as sewers, roads, firefighting arrangements, banks (as we are yet again reminded), and, so very recently, the Internet. No romantic, Hume realized that trust will not exist unless there is some sort of enforcement of the rules of the game, because even a conscientious person will realize that if others break the rules, then his own conformity would impoverish him while others prosper. Anticipating the phenomenon known from ecologist Garrett Hardin's famous 1968 paper as "the tragedy of the commons," Hume recognized that trust at the cultural level has enormous benefits, but is a complicated, cultural-cooperation phenomenon. For one thing, it requires cultural solutions to the problem of ensuring adherence to the rule whereby all do fairly well and but none does so well as to endanger the common resource.

Many pressing moral problems of our time are problems about how best to regulate certain practices, organizations, and institutions, how best to solve problems at the global rather than the local level, how best to achieve sustainability. Many social scientists as well as journalists, those in government, and ordinary thoughtful citizens, are gathering data and working to understand where a policy has gone wrong, and how to put it right. Human cultures have become so complex that even understanding some small part, such as the criminal law of a single country, is a vast undertaking.

Consider just one example: what kind of regulations should govern stem cell research? To begin to make progress on that question, one has to know quite a lot of science—what stem cells are, what about them makes them suitable for medical research and therapy, what diseases might be addressed using stem cell research, and what objections might be raised against it. For a completely different example, what regulations should govern the hunting of wolves? What regulations should govern drugs such as marijuana, cocaine, and heroin? How much religious tolerance is too much? For any of these matters, knowledge is always preferable to ignorance; there is always an awesome amount to know; and for our culture, one of the biggest issues concerns whom to trust in the knowledge domain. To answer this, you have to know *something* in order to have a reasonable belief about who is likely to be trustworthy for the technical details.

Notes

1. Introduction

1. Edwin McAmis augmented my knowledge of legal history by pointing out that English justice acquired its distinguishing characteristics only after the Norman Conquest of 1066. At first the Normans did nothing to change Anglo-Saxon trial by ordeal. Indeed, they introduced their own God-dependent variation—trial by battle. All that changed soon after Henry II came to the throne in 1154. Henry learned that many formerly royal lands scattered throughout England were now possessed by others. The violence, even anarchy, that bedeviled the reign of King Stephen, Henry's predecessor, may have occasioned much of this attrition. Were those currently in possession of these lands squatters, or had they received some benefice from a former monarch? The question was not easily answered because the English government did not bother to create and maintain a record of its own acts until well after 1200.

King Henry did not intend to brawl for land. He introduced a method of dispute resolution, well recognized in Normandy at that time but unknown in England. The king ordered the sheriff of each shire where contested land was located to assemble a group of twelve men to decide whose rights to each piece of land were superior. Those selected had to be locals who knew facts about the possession of the land at relevant dates. Those called met and decided who had the better claim to possess a given piece of land. Whichever way the decision went, King Henry accepted the results so long as the decision was agreed unanimously.

This method worked well enough so that Henry's barons, who had the same problems, asked him for permission to use the identical procedure. The king issued writs to any sheriff on their behalf upon payment of a fee to the royal treasury. Thereafter other people began to request writs to resolve many kinds of controversies. In this way, royal administration of justice came to England. Before that time, justice had been administered by the shire, the hundred, or the manor. The king was thought to have no part in it. In time royal courts were established and royal judges declared *common law* (i.e., law common to everyone in England).

This was the beginning of the English jury. At first, the neighbors had to know the facts and no testimony was taken in court. Another couple of hundred years passed before it became standard practice to ask jurors to determine facts based on what they heard and saw in court rather than upon their own knowledge.

2. See this point affirmed by Philip Kitcher, "Biology and Ethics," in *The Oxford Handbook of Ethics*, ed. D. Copp (Oxford: Oxford University Press, 2006), 163–85; and by Catherine Wilson, "The Biological Basis and Ideational Superstructure of Ethics," *Canadian Journal of Philosophy* 26 (supplement) (2002): 211–44. What Hume actually said was more nuanced than legend has it:

> In every system of morality, which I have hitherto met with, I have always remark'd, that the author proceeds for some time in the ordinary way of reasoning, and establishes the being of a God, or makes observations concerning human affairs; when of a sudden I am surpriz'd to find, that instead of the usual copulations of propositions, *is*, and *is not*, I meet with no proposition that is not connected with an *ought*, or an *ought not*. This change is imperceptible; but is, however, of the last consequence. For as this *ought*, or *ought not*, expresses some new relation or affirmation, 'tis necessary that it should be observ'd and explain'd; and at the same time that a reason shou'd be given, for what seems altogether inconceivable, how this new relation can be a deduction from others, which are entirely different from it.

David Hume, *A Treatise of Human Nature*, ed. David Fate Norton and Mary J. Norton (Oxford: Oxford University Press, 2000), 3.1.1.27.

3. David Hume, *A Treatise of Human Nature*, 2.3.3.4.

4. Simon Blackburn, "Response to Marc Hauser's Princeton Tanner Lecture," unpublished manuscript, 2008, available at http://www.phil.cam.ac.uk/~swb24/PAPERS/Hauser.pdf.

5. Simon Blackburn, *How to Read Hume* (London: Granta, 2008).

6. As Annette Baier has pointed out, "*The Treatise* used reflection first to destroy one version of reason, then to establish the sort of customs, habits, abilities and passions that can bear their own moral survey." See Annette Baier, *A Progress of Sentiments: Reflections on Hume's Treatise* (Cambridge, MA: Harvard University Press, 1991), 288.

7. See chapters 7 and 8.

8. Paul Thagard and Karsten Verbeurgt, "Coherence as Constraint Satisfaction," *Cognitive Science* 22, no. 1: 1–24.

9. See James Woodward, "Interventionist Theories of Causation in Psychological Perspective," in *Causal Learning: Psychology, Philosophy and Computation*, ed. A. Gopnik and L. Schulz (New York: Oxford University Press, 2007),19–36.

10. David Danks, "The Psychology of Causal Perception and Reasoning," in *The Oxford Handbook of Causation*, ed. H. Beebee, C. Hitchcock, and P. Menzies (Oxford: Oxford University Press, 2009), 447–70.

11. I realized only recently that "kith" is not a very common word in U.S. vernacular. It means relatives, friends, and others in the clan or community. But it *is* useful, and so I wish to use it.

12. See also James Woodward and John Allman, "Moral Intuition: Its Neural Substrates and Normative Significance," *Journal of Physiology–Paris* 101, no. 4–6 (2007): 179–202; Alex Mesoudi, "How Cultural Evolutionary Theory Can Inform Social Psychology and Vice Versa," *Psychological Review*, no. 116: 929–52 (2009).

13. See Alasdair MacIntyre's book *After Virtue* (Notre Dame, IN: University of Notre Dame Press, 2007) for a wonderful discussion of the history of the various ways that morals, values, virtues, and ethics have been understood. The current way within western cultures is certainly not the only way.

14. Mark Johnson, *Moral Imagination: Implications of Cognitive Science for Ethics* (Chicago: University of Chicago Press, 1993).

15. Eytan Avital and Eva Jablonka, *Animal Traditions: Behavioural Inheritance in Evolution* (New York: Cambridge University Press, 2000); Robert Boyd and Peter J. Richerson, "Solving the Puzzle of Human Cooperation," in *Evolution and Culture*, ed. Stephen C. Levinson (Cambridge, MA: MIT Press, 2005); Peter J. Richerson and Robert Boyd, *Not by Genes Alone: How Culture Transformed Human Evolution* (Chicago: University of Chicago Press, 2005).

16. *Hominins* are defined in terms of the last common ancestor of modern humans (*Homo sapiens sapiens*) and all those extinct species in the Homo subfamily, including *Homo erectus, Homo habilis, Homo rudolfensis, Homo ergaster, Homo floresiensis, Homo heidelbergensis,* and *Homo neanderthalensis,* as well as some nine or ten transitional hominins. For a concise overview, see Bernard A. Wood, *Human Evolution: A Very Short Introduction* (Oxford: Oxford University Press, 2005); Chad E. Forbes and Jordan Grafman, "The Role of the Prefrontal Cortex in Social Cognition and Moral Judgment". *Annual Review of Neuroscience* no.33 (2010): 299–324.

17. To borrow a phrase coined by the late neuroscientist Paul MacLean. See, for example, Paul D. MacLean, *The Triune Brain in Evolution: Role in Paleocerebral Functions* (New York: Plenum Press, 1990).

2. Brain-Based Values

1. See also Owen J. Flanagan, *The Really Hard Problem: Meaning in a Material World* (Cambridge, MA: MIT Press, 2007). See especially chapter 4.

2. C. Sue Carter, James Harris, and Stephen W. Porges, "Neural and Evolutionary Perspectives on Empathy," in *The Social Neuroscience of Empathy*, ed. J. Decety and W. Ickes (Cambridge, MA: MIT Press, 2009), 169–82.

3. Eric B. Keverne, "Understanding Well-Being in the Evolutionary Context of Brain Development," *Philosophical Transactions of the Royal Society of London B: Biological Sciences* 359, no. 1449 (2004): 1349–58.

It may be that parental and mate care arose in mammals and birds by convergent evolution, but as Ralph Greenspan pointed out to me, it may be that there was a common ancestor who cared for its young. See Qingjin Meng et al., "Palaeontology: Parental Care in an Ornithischian Dinosaur," *Nature* 431, no. 7005 (2004): 145–46.

4. Jaak Panksepp, "Feeling the Pain of Social Loss," *Science* 302, no. 5643 (2003): 237–39. Note, however, that alligators will defend the nest if the young squeal. Synapsids, or reptile-like mammals, are believed to have branched off from sauropsids (reptiles) about 315 million years ago. Little is known about the evolution of mammals because mammals are the only surviving direct descendants of synapsids, all other intermediate species having become extinct.

5. I mention this because some clinical psychologists have a rather different use of *attachment*.

6. L. Vigilant et al., "African Populations and the Evolution of Human Mitochondrial DNA," *Science* 253, no. 5027 (1991): 1503–7.

7. Christopher S. Henshilwood et al., "An Early Bone Tool Industry from the Middle Stone Age at Blombos Cave, South Africa: Implications for the Origins of Modern Human Behaviour, Symbolism and Language," *Journal of Human Evolution* 41, no. 6 (2001): 631–78; Christopher Henshilwood et al., "Middle Stone Age Shell Beads from South Africa," *Science* 304: 404.

8. Sally McBrearty and Alison S. Brooks, "The Revolution That Wasn't: A New Interpretation of the Origin of Modern Human Behavior," *Journal of Human Evolution* 39, no. 5 (2000): 453–563.

9. Curtis W. Marean, "When the Sea Saved Humanity," *Scientific American* 303 (2010): 55–61.

10. See again Marean, "When the Sea Saved Humanity."

11. Susan Neiman, *Moral Clarity: A Guide for Grown-up Idealists* (Orlando, FL: Harcourt, 2008).

12. Angie A. Kehagia, Graham K. Murray, and Trevor W. Robbins, "Learning and Cognitive Flexibility: Frontostriatal Function and Monoaminergic Modulation," *Current Opinion in Neurobiology* 20, no. 2 (2010): 199–204; Derek E. Lyons, Andrew G. Young, and Frank C. Keil, "The Hidden Structure of Overimitation," *Proceedings of the National Academy of Sciences* 104, no. 50 (2007): 19751–56.

13. Ian J. Deary, Lars Penke, and Wendy Johnson, "The Neuroscience of Human Intelligence Differences," *Nature Reviews Neuroscience* 11, no. 3 (2010): 201–11.

14. T. W. Robbins and A.F.T. Arnsten, "The Neuropsychopharmacology of Fronto-Executive Function: Monoaminergic Modulation," *Annual Review of Neuroscience* 32, no. 1 (2009): 267–87.

15. Matt Ridley, *The Rational Optimist* (New York: Harper Collins, 2010).

16. Roy F. Baumeister, *The Cultural Animal Human Nature, Meaning, and Social Life* (New York: Oxford University Press, 2005); Ernst Fehr and Simon Gächter, "Cooperation and Punishment in Public Goods Experiments," *American Economic Review* 90 (2000): 980–94; Herbert Gintis, *The Bounds of Reason: Game Theory and the Unification of the Behavioral Sciences* (Princeton: Princeton University Press, 2009); Sarah Blaffer Hrdy, *Mother Nature: A History of Mothers, Infants, and Natural Selection* (New York: Pantheon Books, 1999); Richard E. Nisbett and Dov Cohen, *Culture of Honor: The Psychology of Violence in the South* (Boulder, CO: Westview Press, 1996); Peter J. Richerson, Robert Boyd, and Joseph Henrich, "Gene-Culture Coevolution in the Age of Genomics," *Proceedings of the National Academy of Sciences* 107, Supplement 2 (2010): 8985–92.

17. Avital and Jablonka, *Animal Traditions*; Gregory Cochran and Henry Harpending, *The 10,000 Year Explosion: How Civilization Accelerated Human Evolution* (New York: Basic Books, 2009).

18. Avital and Jablonka, *Animal Traditions*.

19. It is not yet settled whether the genetic changes came first, and made drinking camel and cow milk advantageous, or whether dairying preceded the genetic changes, perhaps as a way of adding to mother's milk, and the genetic changes followed.

20. David Danks, "Constraint-Based Human Causal Learning," in *Proceedings of the 6th International Conference on Cognitive Modeling (ICCM-2004)*, ed. M. Lovett, C. Schunn, C. Lebiere, and P. Munro (Mahwah, NJ: Lawrence Erlbaum Associates, 2004): 342–43.

21. See Patricia S. Churchland, "Inference to the Best Decision," in *The Oxford Handbook of Philosophy and Neuroscience*, ed. John Bickle (New York: Oxford University Press, 2009), 419–30. See also Deborah Talmi et al., "How Humans Integrate the Prospects of Pain and Reward During Choice," *Journal of Neuroscience* 29, no. 46 (2009): 14617–26.

22. Matthew Gervais and David Sloan Wilson, "The Evolution and Functions of Laughter and Humor: A Synthetic Approach," *Quarterly Review of Biology* 80, no. 4 (2005): 395–430.

23. Robert M. Sapolsky, *A Primate's Memoir* (New York: Scribner, 2001).

24. See Christine M. Korsgaard, *The Sources of Normativity* (New York: Cambridge University Press, 1996).

25. See Amanda M. Seed, Nicola S. Clayton, and Nathan J. Emery, "Postconflict Third-Party Affiliation in Rooks, *Corvus frugilegus*," *Current Biology* 17, no. 2 (2007): 152–58.

26. G. Cordoni and E. Palagi, "Reconciliation in Wolves (*Canis lupus*): New Evidence for a Comparative Perspective," *Ethology* 114, no. 3 (2008): 298–308.

3. Caring and Caring For

1. Many bird species are also highly social, and what is known so far about their homologue of oxytocin, mesotocin, indicates that it plays a role in offspring and mate attachment similar to that of oxytocin in mammals. Some differences in mechanisms are likely, since the common ancestor of mammals and birds lived about 300 million years ago, and the brains of birds are organized very differently from those of mammals. My discussion in this book will focus only on mammalian nervous systems, where much more is known, but from time to time, I will make observations about bird sociality. On bird sociality, see Nicola S. Clayton, Joanna M. Dally, and Nathan J. Emery, "Social Cognition by Food-Caching Corvids: The Western Scrub-Jay as a Natural Psychologist," *Philosophical Transactions of the Royal Society B: Biological Sciences* 362, no. 1480 (2007): 507–22; James L. Goodson, "The Vertebrate Social Behavior Network: Evolutionary Themes and Variations," *Hormones and Behavior* 48, no. 1 (2005): 11–22; and James L. Goodson et al., "Mesotocin and Nonapeptide Receptors Promote Estrildid Flocking Behavior," *Science* 325 (2009): 862–66; as well as Jaak Panksepp, *Affective Neuroscience: The Foundations of Human and Animal Emotions* (New York: Oxford University Press, 1998).

2. Panksepp, *Affective Neuroscience*. Antonio R. Damasio, *The Feeling of What Happens: Body and Emotion in the Making of Consciousness* (New York: Harcourt Brace, 1999).

3. A. D. Craig, "A New View of Pain as a Homeostatic Emotion," *Trends in Neurosciences* 26, no. 6 (2003): 303–7; Craig, "Pain Mechanisms: Labeled Lines versus Convergence in Central Processing," *Annual Review of Neuroscience* 26, no. 1 (2003): 1–30.

4. A. D. Craig, "How Do You Feel? Interoception: The Sense of the Physiological Condition of the Body," *Nature Reviews Neuroscience* 3, no. 8 (2002): 655–66; Rodolfo R. Llinás, *I of the Vortex: From Neurons to Self* (Cambridge, MA: MIT Press, 2001); Damasio, *The Feeling of What Happens*; Panksepp, *Affective Neuroscience*.

5. Antonio R. Damasio, *Self Comes to Mind: Constructing the Conscious Brain* (New York: Knopf/Pantheon, 2010).

6. Yawei Cheng et al., "Love Hurts: An fMRI Study," *Neuroimage* 51, no. 2 (2010): 923–29.

7. This is perhaps what Hume had in mind when he used the expression *moral sentiment*. See Blackburn, *How to Read Hume*.

8. Stephen W. Porges and C. Sue Carter, "Neurobiology and Evolution: Mechanisms, Mediators, and Adaptive Consequences of Caregiving," in *Self Interest and Beyond: Toward a New Understanding of Human Caregiving*, ed. S. L. Brown, R. M. Brown, and L. A. Penner (Oxford: Oxford University Press, in press). See also Eric B. Keverne, "Genomic Imprinting and the Evolution of Sex Differences in Mammalian Reproductive Strategies," *Advances in Genetics* 59 (2007): 217–43.

9. Porges and Carter, Neurobiology and Evolution."

10. Quoted in Elizabeth Pennisi, "On the Origin of Cooperation," *Science* 325, no. 5945 (2009): 1196–99.

11. Keverne, "Genomic Imprinting and the Evolution of Sex Differences."

12. For a wonderful account of this, see Donald W. Pfaff, *The Neuroscience of Fair Play: Why We (Usually) Follow the Golden Rule* (New York: Dana Press, 2007).

13. K. D. Broad, J. P. Curley, and E. B. Keverne, "Mother-Infant Bonding and the Evolution of Mammalian Social Relationships," *Philosophical Transactions of the Royal Society B: Biological Sciences* 361, no. 1476 (2006): 2199–214.

14. Eric B. Keverne, "Understanding Well-Being in the Evolutionary Context of Brain Development," *Philosophical Transactions of the Royal Society of London B: Biological Sciences* 359, no. 1449 (2004): 1349–58.

15. Kathleen C. Light et al., "Deficits in Plasma Oxytocin Responses and Increased Negative Affect, Stress, and Blood Pressure in Mothers with Cocaine Exposure During Pregnancy," *Addictive Behaviors* 29, no. 8 (2004): 1541–64.

16. See Don M. Tucker, Phan Luu, and Douglas Derryberry, "Love Hurts: The Evolution of Empathic Concern through the Encephalization of Nociceptive Capacity," *Development and Psychopathology* 17, no. 3 (2005): 699–713; Cheng et al., "Love Hurts: An fMRI Study."

17. A. D. Craig, K. Krout, and E. T. Zhang, "Cortical Projections of VMpo, a Specific Pain and Temperature Relay in Primate Thalamus," *Abstracts—Society for Neuroscience* 21 (1995): 1165.

18. Georg F. Striedter, "Précis of *Principles of Brain Evolution*," *Behavioral and Brain Sciences* 29, no. 1 (2006): 1–12.

19. A. D. Craig, "Pain Mechanisms: Labeled Lines versus Convergence in Central Processing," *Annual Review of Neuroscience* 26, no. 1 (2003): 1–30.

20. A. D. Craig, "Interoception and Emotion: A Neuroanatomical Perspective," in *Handbook of Emotions*, 3rd ed., ed. Michael Lewis, Jeannette M. Haviland-Jones, and Lisa F. Barrett (New York: Guilford, 2008), 272–88.

21. A. D. Craig, "How Do You Feel—Now? The Anterior Insula and Human Awareness," *Nature Reviews Neuroscience* 10, no. 1 (2009): 59–70.

22. See Damasio, *The Feeling of What Happens*. On the role of fear, see Pfaff, *The Neuroscience of Fair Play*.

23. Naomi I. Eisenberger and Matthew D. Lieberman, "Why Rejection Hurts: A Common Neural Alarm System for Physical and Social Pain," *Trends in Cognitive Sciences* 8, no. 7 (2004): 294–300.

24. See Robert D. Hare, *Without Conscience: The Disturbing World of the Psychopaths among Us* (New York: Pocket Books, 1993); Martha Stout, *The Sociopath Next Door: The Ruthless versus the Rest of Us* (New York: Broadway Books, 2005).

25. Robert D. Hare, *Manual for the Hare Psychopathy Checklist—Revised*, 2nd ed. (Toronto: Multi-Health Systems, 2003); R. D. Hare and C. N. Neumann, "The PCL-R Assessment of Psychopathy: Development, Structural Properties, and New Directions," in *Handbook of Psychopathy*, ed. C. Patrick (New York: Guilford, 2006), 58–88; R.J.R. Blair, "Neuroimaging of Psychopathy and Antisocial Behavior: A Targeted Review," *Current Psychiatry Reports* 12, no. 1 (2010): 76–82. See also my interview (May 2010 in Oxford, England) with Walter Sinnott-Armstrong on The Science Network, http://thesciencenetwork.org/programs/the-rightful-place/the-rightful -place-with-walter-sinnott-armstrong.

26. Kent A. Kiehl, "A Cognitive Neuroscience Perspective on Psychopathy: Evidence for Paralimbic System Dysfunction," *Psychiatry Research* 142 (2006): 107–28.

27. A. Raine et al., "Hippocampal Structural Asymmetry in Unsuccessful Psychopaths," *Biological Psychiatry* 552 (2004): 185–91.

28. T. D. Gunter, M. G. Vaughn, and R. A. Philibert, "Behavioral Genetics in Antisocial Spectrum Disorders and Psychopathy: A Review of the Recent Literature," *Behavioral Sciences & the Law* 28, no. 2 (2010): 148–73.

29. See "Acquiring a Conscience" in chapter 6.

30. Todd M. Preuss, "Evolutionary Specializations of Primate Brain Systems," in *Primate Origins and Adaptations*, ed. M. J. Ravoso and M. Dagosto (New York: Kluwer Academic/Plenum Press: 2007), 625–75.

31. Sara Jahfari et al., "Responding with Restraint: What Are the Neurocognitive Mechanisms?" *Journal of Cognitive Neuroscience* 22, no. 7 (2010): 1479–92; Caroline H. Williams-Gray et al., "Catechol O-Methyltransferase Val[158]met Genotype Influences Frontoparietal Activity During Planning in Patients with Parkinson's Disease," *Journal of Neuroscience* 27, no. 18 (2007): 4832–38; S. E. Winder-Rhodes et al., "Effects of Modafinil and Prazosin on Cognitive and Physiological Functions in Healthy Volunteers," *Journal of Psychopharmacology* (in press).

32. Johnson, *Moral Imagination*.

33. Stephen W. Porges, "The Polyvagal Perspective," *Biological Psychology* 74, no. 2 (2007): 116–43.

34. Panksepp, *Affective Neuroscience*, chapter 13, "Love and the Social Bond: The Brain Sources of Sorrow and Grief."

35. Broad, Curley, and Keverne, "Mother-Infant Bonding."

36. Llinás, *I of the Vortex*.

37. See Preuss, "Evolutionary Specializations of Primate Brain Systems," and for a more technical discussion, Preuss, "Primate Brain Evoution in Phylogenetic Context," in *Evolution of Nervous Systems: A Comprehensive Reference*, vol. 4, ed. Jon H. Kaas and Todd M. Preuss (Amsterdam: Academic Press, 2007), 1–34.

38. Tucker, Luu, and Derryberry, "Love Hurts."

39. Christian Keysers and David I. Perrett, "Demystifying Social Cognition: A Hebbian Perspective," *Trends in Cognitive Sciences* 8, no. 11 (2004): 501–7.

49. See Clayton, Dally, and Emery, "Social Cognition by Food-Caching Corvids."

41. Leah Krubitzer, "The Magnificent Compromise: Cortical Field Evolution in Mammals," *Neuron* 56 (2007): 201–9.

42. Panksepp, *Affective Neuroscience*, chapter 13.

43. Devra G. Kleiman, "Monogamy in Mammals," *Quarterly Review of Biology* 52, no. 1 (1977): 39–69.

44. Ibid.

45. The measure of depression in voles, for example, involves seeing how vigorously they swim when dropped in a pail of water, or how vigorous or indifferent their hedonic response is when given a sweet to lick.

46. See Lisa Belkin, "The Evolution of Dad," *New York Times Magazine*, June 16, 2010; also at http://parenting.blogs.nytimes.com/2010/06/16/the-evolution-of-dad/.

47. Jacqueline M. Bishop, Colleen O'Ryan, and Jennifer U. M. Jarvis, "Social Common Mole-Rats Enhance Outbreeding Via Extra-Pair Mating," *Biology Letters* 3, no. 2 (2007): 176–79; Aurélie Cohas and Dominique Allainé, "Social Structure Influences Extra-Pair Paternity in Socially Monogamous Mammals," *Biology Letters* 5, no. 3 (2009): 313–16.

48. Eric B. Keverne, "Reproductive Behaviour," in *Reproduction in Mammals*, vol. 4: *Reproductive Fitness*, ed. C. R. Austin and R. V. Short (Cambridge: Cambridge University Press, 1984), 133–75; Keverne, "Central Mechanisms Underlying the Neural and Neuroendocrine Determinants of Maternal Behaviour," *Psychoneuroendocrinology* 13, no. 1–2 (1988): 127–41; Keverne and K. M. Kendrick, "Neurochemical Changes Accompanying Parturition and Their Significance for Maternal Behavior," in *Mammalian Parenting: Biochemical, Neurobiological and Behavioral Determinants*, ed. N. A. Krasnegor and R. S. Bridges (New York: Oxford University Press, 1990), 281–304.

49. See this insight well discussed in Porges and Carter, "Neurobiology and Evolution."

50. Michael R. Murphy et al., "Changes in Oxytocin and Vasopressin Secretion During Sexual Activity in Men," *The Journal of Clinical Endocrinology & Metabolism* 65, no. 4 (1987): 738–41.

51. A. Courtney DeVries et al., "Corticotropin-Releasing Factor Induces Social Preferences in Male Prairie Voles," *Psychoneuroendocrinology* 27, no. 6 (2002): 705–14.

52. K. L. Bales et al., "Neonatal Oxytocin Manipulations Have Long-Lasting, Sexually Dimorphic Effects on Vasopressin Receptors," *Neuroscience* 144, no. 1 (2007): 38–45; Janet K. Bester-Meredith and Catherine A. Marler, "Vasopressin and Aggression in Cross-Fostered California Mice (*Peromyscus californicus*) and White-Footed Mice (*Peromyscus leucopus*)," *Hormones and Behavior* 40, no. 1 (2001): 51–64.

53. Miranda M. Lim, Anne Z. Murphy, and Larry J. Young, "Ventral Striatopallidal Oxytocin and Vasopressin V1a Receptors in the Monogamous Prairie Vole (*Microtus ochrogaster*)," *Journal of Comparative Neurology* 468, no. 4 (2004): 555–70.

54. Zuoxin Wang et al., "Vasopressin in the Forebrain of Common Marmosets (*Callithrix jacchus*): Studies with In Situ Hybridization, Immunocytochemistry and Receptor Autoradiography," *Brain Research* 768, no. 1–2 (1997): 147–56.

55. Karen L. Bales et al., "Oxytocin Has Dose-Dependent Developmental Effects on Pair-Bonding and Alloparental Care in Female Prairie Voles," *Hormones and Behavior* 52, no. 2 (2007): 274–79.

56. Heike Tost et al., "A Common Allele in the Oxytocin Receptor Gene (OXTR) Impacts Prosocial Temperament and Human Hypothalamic-Limbic Structure and Function," *Proceedings of the National Academy of Sciences* 107, no. 31 (2010): 13936–41.

57. Any gene may have two or more alleles, which are differences in the DNA sequence. Since an individual gets one chromosome from each parent, then the gene at a given locus may be the same on both chromosomes (i.e., the alleles are the same), or it may be different (i.e., the alleles are different). Depending on the significance of those differences, there may be trait differences, eye color being one example.

58. The variant of the OXTR gene is known as rs53576A. This was first identified as related to sociality by Sarina M. Rodrigues et al., "Oxytocin Receptor Genetic Variation Relates to Empathy and Stress Reactivity in Humans," *Proceedings of the National Academy of Sciences* 106, no. 50 (2009): 21437–41.

59. G. Domes et al., "Oxytocin Attenuates Amygdala Responses to Emotional Faces Regardless of Valence," *Biological Psychiatry* 62, no. 10 (2007): 1187–90.

69. Frances Champagne and Michael J. Meaney, "Like Mother, Like Daughter: Evidence for Non-Genomic Transmission of Parental Behavior and Stress Responsivity," *Progress in Brain Research* 133 (2001): 287–302; Champagne and Meaney, "Transgenerational Effects of Social Environment on Variations in Maternal Care and Behavioral Response to Novelty," *Behavioral Neuroscience* 121, no. 6 (2007): 1353–63.

61. Michael J. Meaney, "Maternal Care, Gene Expression, and the Transmission of Individual Differences in Stress Reactivity across Generations," *Annual Review of Neuroscience* 24, no. 1 (2003): 1161–92.

62. Dario Maestripieri et al., "Mother-Infant Interactions in Free-Ranging Rhesus Macaques: Relationships between Physiological and Behavioral Variables," *Physiology & Behavior* 96, no. 4–5 (2009): 613–19.

63. Ruth Feldman, Ilanit Gordon, and Orna Zagoory-Sharon, "The Cross-Generation Transmission of Oxytocin in Humans," *Hormones and Behavior* (in press).

64. M. J. Crockett et al., "Serotonin Modulates Behavioral Reactions to Unfairness," *Science* 320, no. 5884 (2008): 1739.

65. There are more types, but these two are probably the only ones relevant here.

66. Jaak Panksepp, "At the Interface of the Affective, Behavioral, and Cognitive Neurosciences: Decoding the Emotional Feelings of the Brain," *Brain and Cognition* 52, no. 1 (2003): 4–14.

67. Jean-Philippe Gouin et al., "Marital Behavior, Oxytocin, Vasopressin, and Wound Healing," *Psychoneuroendocrinology* (in press).

68. Elizabeth A. Phelps et al., "Extinction Learning in Humans: Role of the Amygdala and vmPFC," 43, no. 6 (2004): 897–905; Miranda Olff et al., "A Psychobiological Rationale for Oxytocin in Treatment of Posttraumatic Stress Disorder." *CNS Spectrums* 15, no. 8 (2010): 436–44.

69. Karen L. Bales et al., "Both Oxytocin and Vasopressin May Influence Alloparental Behavior in Male Prairie Voles," *Hormones and Behavior* 45, no. 5 (2004): 354–61.

70. Sabine Fink, Laurent Excoffier, and Gerald Heckel, "Mammalian Monogamy Is Not Controlled by a Single Gene," *Proceedings of the National Academy of Sciences* 103, no. 29 (2006): 10956–60; Leslie M. Turner et al., "Monogamy Evolves through Multiple Mechanisms: Evidence from V1ar in Deer Mice," *Molecular Biology and Evolution* 27, no. 6 (2010): 1269–78.

71. What about *our* genes? Early results from a Swedish study found significant pair-bonding differences between adult human males who carried the "nonmonogamous" variant of the microsatellite region for the AVP receptor (identified in prairie voles but not other monogamous species), and those who did not (see Walum et al., "Genetic Variation in the Vasopressin Receptor 1a Gene (AVPR1A) Associates with Pair-Bonding Behavior in Humans," *Proceedings of the National Academy of Sciences* 105, no. 37 (2008): 14153–56). Intriguing though these results may seem, I must emphasize the qualification "early." Humans, relative to voles, have a truly massive amount of prefrontal territory, and as noted, this allows for tremendous flexibility and variability in human behavior, including variability owed to learned cultural norms and expectations. Humans are susceptible to cultural and environmental influences, and roughly 80% of cortical growth and change takes place after birth. Gene-environment interactions, along with gene-gene interactions, means that assumptions about "the gene for monogamy" oversimplify to the point of futility. (See chapter 4 for more on gene-behavior relationships.)

72. George P. Murdock and Suzanne F. Wilson, "Settlement Patterns and Community Organization: Cross-Cultural Codes 3," *Ethnology* 11 (1972): 254–95.

73. L. Fortunato and M. Archetti, "Evolution of Monogamous Marriage by Maximization of Inclusive Fitness," *Journal of Evolutionary Biology* 23, no. 1 (2010): 149–56.

74. Chad E. Forbes and Jordan Grafman, "The Role of the Human Prefrontal Cortex in Social Cognition and Moral Judgment," *Annual Review of Neuroscience* 33, no. 1 (2010): 299–324.

75. Richard E. Nisbett, *The Geography of Thought: How Asians and Westerners Think Differently—and Why* (New York: Free Press, 2003); Nisbett and Cohen, *Culture of Honor.*

76. See Richerson and Boyd, *Not by Genes Alone*, which emphasizes the role of imitation, and contrast this with Christine A. Caldwell and Ailsa E. Millen, "Social Learning Mechanisms and Cumulative Cultural Evolution" (*Psychological Science* 20, no. 12 [2009]: 1478–83), which suggests the case is by no means closed.

77. Ann M. Graybiel, "Habits, Rituals, and the Evaluative Brain," *Annual Review of Neuroscience* 31(2008): 359–87.

78. Benjamin Kilham and Ed Gray, *Among the Bears: Raising Orphan Cubs in the Wild* (New York: Henry Holt, 2002).

4. Cooperating and Trusting

1. See also Avital and Jablonka, *Animal Traditions*.

2. Julianne Holt-Lunstad, Wendy A. Birmingham, and Kathleen C. Light, "Influence of a 'Warm Touch' Support Enhancement Intervention among Married Couples on Ambulatory Blood Pressure, Oxytocin, Alpha Amylase, and Cortisol," *Psychosomatic Medicine* 70, no. 9 (2008): 976–85.

3. Richerson and Boyd, *Not by Genes Alone*.

4. F. Boas, *The Central Eskimo* (Lincoln: University of Nebraska Press, 1888/1964).

5. Joseph Henrich et al., "Markets, Religion, Community Size, and the Evolution of Fairness and Punishment," *Science* 327, no. 5972 (2010): 1480–84.

6. Daniel Friedman, *Morals and Markets: An Evolutionary Account of the Modern World* (New York: Palgrave Macmillan, 2008).

7. Adam Powell, Stephen Shennan, and Mark G. Thomas, "Late Pleistocene Demography and the Appearance of Modern Human Behavior," *Science* 324, no. 5932 (2009): 1298–301; Michelle A. Kline and Robert Boyd, "Population Size Predicts Technological Complexity in Oceania," *Proceedings of the Royal Society B: Biological Sciences* 277, no. 1693 (2010): 2559–64.

8. Henrich et al., "Markets, Religion, Community Size, and the Evolution of Fairness and Punishment."

9. David Remnick, *Lenin's Tomb: The Last Days of the Soviet Empire* (New York: Random House, 1993).

10. These definitions are drawn from a useful paper by S. A. West, C. El Mouden, and A. Gardner, "16 Common Misconceptions about the Evolution of Cooperation in Humans," *Evolution and Human Behavior* (in press); http://www.zoo.ox.ac.uk/group/west/pdf/West_etal.pdf.

11. Susan Perry et al., "White-faced Capuchins Cooperate to Rescue a Groupmate from a *Boa constrictor*." *Folia Primatologica* 74 (2003): 109–11.

12. Ming Zhang and Jing-Xia Cai, "Neonatal Tactile Stimulation Enhances Spatial Working Memory, Prefrontal Long-Term Potentiation, and D1 Receptor Activation in Adult Rats," *Neurobiology of Learning and Memory* 89, no. 4 (2008): 397–406. See also Champagne and Meaney, "Like Mother, Like Daughter."

13. R.I.M. Dunbar, "Coevolution of Neocortical Size, Group Size and Language in Humans," *Behavioral and Brain Sciences* 16, no. 4 (1993): 681–94; R.I.M. Dunbar, *Grooming, Gossip and the Evolution of Language* (London: Faber and Faber, 1996).

14. Scott Creel and Nancy Marusha Creel, "Communal Hunting and Pack Size in African Wild Dogs, *Lycaon pictus*," *Animal Behaviour* 50, no. 5 (1995): 1325–39.

15. But see two magnificent books: *Mind of the Raven* (New York: Cliff Street Books, 1999) and *One Man's Owl* (Princeton, NJ: Princeton University Press, 1987), both by Bernd Heinrich.

16. Christophe Boesch et al., "Altruism in Forest Chimpanzees: The Case of Adoption," *PLoS ONE* 5, no. 1 (2010): e8901.

17. Natalie Vasey, "The Breeding System of Wild Red Ruffed Lemurs (*Varecia rubra*): A Preliminary Report," *Primates* 48, no. 1 (2007): 41–54.

18. Marc Bekoff and Jessica Pierce, *Wild Justice: The Moral Lives of Animals* (Chicago: University of Chicago Press, 2009), 56.

19. Mietje Germonpré et al., "Fossil Dogs and Wolves from Palaeolithic Sites in Belgium, the Ukraine and Russia: Osteometry, Ancient DNA and Stable Isotopes," *Journal of Archaeological Science* 36, no. 2 (2009): 473–90.

20. W. Hoesch, "Uber Ziegen hutende Bärenpaviane (*Papio ursinus ruacana*)," *Zeitschrift für Tierpsychologie* 18 (1961): 297–301. From Dorothy L. Cheney and Robert M. Seyfarth, *Baboon Metaphysics: The Evolution of a Social Mind* (Chicago: University of Chicago Press, 2007).

21. M. Kosfeld et al., "Oxytocin Increases Trust in Humans," *Nature* 435, no. 7042 (2005): 673–76.

22. B. King-Casas et al., "The Rupture and Repair of Cooperation in Borderline Personality Disorder," *Science* 321, no. 5890 (2008): 806–10.

23. Carsten K. W. De Dreu et al., "The Neuropeptide Oxytocin Regulates Parochial Altruism in Intergroup Conflict among Humans," *Science* 328, no. 5984 (2010): 1408–11.

24. P. J. Zak, A. A. Stanton, and S. Ahmadi, "Oxytocin Increases Generosity in Humans," *PLoS ONE* 2, no. 11 (2007): e1128.

25. Panksepp, *Affective Neuroscience*; Tucker, Luu, and Derryberry, "Love Hurts."

26. Gregor Domes et al., "Oxytocin Improves 'Mind-Reading' in Humans," *Biological Psychiatry* 61, no. 6 (2007): 731–33. The test is available online at http://www.questionwritertracker.com/index.php/quiz/display?id=61&token=Z4MK3TB.

27. P. Kirsch et al., "Oxytocin Modulates Neural Circuitry for Social Cognition and Fear in Humans," *Journal of Neuroscience* 25, no. 49 (2005): 11489–93.

28. Gregor Domes et al., "Effects of Intranasal Oxytocin on Emotional Face Processing in Women," *Psychoneuroendocrinology* 35, no. 1 (2010): 83–93.

29. R. R. Thompson et al., "Sex-Specific Influences of Vasopressin on Human Social Communication," *Proceedings of the National Academy of Sciences* 103, no. 20 (2006): 7889–94.

30. S. E. Taylor et al., "Biobehavioral Responses to Stress in Females: Tend-and-Befriend, Not Fight-or-Flight," *Psychological Review* 107, no. 3 (2000): 411–29.

31. See, for example, Karen L. Bales et al., "Effects of Stress on Parental Care Are Sexually Dimorphic in Prairie Voles," *Physiology & Behavior* 87, no. 2 (2006): 424–29.

32. C. Sue Carter et al., "Oxytocin, Vasopressin and Sociality," in *Progress in Brain Research 170: Advances in Vasopressin and Oxytocin: From Genes to Behaviour*

to Disease, ed. Inga D. Neumann and Rainer Landgraf (New York: Elsevier, 2008), 331–36. See also Louann Brizendine, *The Female Brain* (New York: Morgan Road Books, 2006), and *The Male Brain* (New York: Broadway Books, 2010).

33. Just go to Google and enter the search phrase "buy oxytocin."

34. Bales et al., "Oxytocin Has Dose-Dependent Developmental Effects."

35. See the editorial "Extending Trust," *Nature Neuroscience* 13, no. 8 (2010): 905.

36. Thomas Baumgartner et al., "Oxytocin Shapes the Neural Circuitry of Trust and Trust Adaptation in Humans," *Neuron* 58, no. 4 (2008): 639–50.

37. Eric Hollander et al., "Oxytocin Increases Retention of Social Cognition in Autism," *Biological Psychiatry* 61 (2007): 498–503.

38. Elissar Andari et al., "Promoting Social Behavior with Oxytocin in High-Functioning Autism Spectrum Disorders," *Proceedings of the National Academy of Sciences* 107, no. 9 (2010): 4389–94.

39. Katherine E. Tansey et al., "Oxytocin Receptor (OXTR) Does Not Play a Major Role in the Aetiology of Autism: Genetic and Molecular Studies," *Neuroscience Letters* 474, no. 3 (2010): 163–67. For a review, see Thomas R. Insel, "The Challenge of Translation in Social Neuroscience: A Review of Oxytocin, Vasopressin, and Affiliative Behavior," *Neuron* 65, no. 6 (2010): 768–79.

40. C. Heim et al., "Lower CSF Oxytocin Concentrations in Women with a History of Childhood Abuse," *Molecular Psychiatry* 14, no. 10 (2008): 954–58.

41. Olff et al., "A Psychobiological Rationale for Oxytocin in Treatment of Post-traumatic Stress Disorder."

42. Insel, "The Challenge of Translation in Social Neuroscience."

43. This section is based on a collaboration between Christopher Suhler and me, and is drawn from our forthcoming paper, "The Neurobiological Basis of Morality," in *The Oxford Handbook of Neuroethics*, ed. Judy Illes and Barbara J. Sahakian (Oxford: Oxford University Press, in press).

44. Robert L. Trivers, "The Evolution of Reciprocal Altruism," *Quarterly Review of Biology* 46, no. 1 (1971): 35.

45. Bekoff and Pierce, *Wild Justice*, chapter 2.

46. Marc D. Hauser, "Costs of Deception: Cheaters Are Punished in Rhesus Monkeys (*Macaca mulatta*)," *Proceedings of the National Academy of Sciences of the United States of America* 89, no. 24 (1992): 12137–39.

47. Tim Clutton-Brock, "Cooperation between Non-Kin in Animal Societies," *Nature* 462, no. 7269 (2009): 51–57.

48. Ernst Fehr and Simon Gächter, "Cooperation and Punishment in Public Goods Experiments."

49. Ernst Fehr and Simon Gächter, "Altruistic Punishment in Humans," *Nature* 415, no. 6868 (2002): 137–40.

50. See Ernst Fehr and Urs Fischbacher, "Third-Party Punishment and Social Norms," *Evolution and Human Behavior* 25, no. 2 (2004): 63–87.

51. Fehr and Gächter, "Altruistic Punishment in Humans," 139.

52. See Peggy La Cerra and Roger Bingham, *The Origin of Minds: Evolution, Uniqueness, and the New Science of the Self* (New York: Harmony Books, 2002);

M. Milinski, D. Semmann, and H. J. Krambeck, "Reputation Helps Solve the 'Tragedy of the Commons,'" *Nature* 415, no. 6870 (2002): 424–26.

53. For a useful collection on cooperation, see Herbert Gintis et al., *Moral Sentiments and Material Interests: The Foundations of Cooperation in Economic Life* (Cambridge, MA: MIT Press, 2004).

54. Bettina Rockenbach and Manfred Milinski, "The Efficient Interaction of Indirect Reciprocity and Costly Punishment," *Nature* 444, no. 7120 (2006): 718–23.

55. Ibid.

56. Jorge M. Pacheco, Francisco C. Santos, and Fabio A.C.C. Chalub, "Stern-Judging: A Simple, Successful Norm Which Promotes Cooperation under Indirect Reciprocity," *PLoS Computational Biology* 2, no. 12 (2006): e178.

57. Brian Hare et al., "Tolerance Allows Bonobos to Outperform Chimpanzees on a Cooperative Task," *Current Biology* 17, no. 7 (2007): 619–23.

58. See also Alicia P. Melis, Brian Hare, and Michael Tomasello, "Engineering Cooperation in Chimpanzees: Tolerance Constraints on Cooperation," *Animal Behaviour* 72, no. 2 (2006): 275–86.

59. On the other hand, in field studies, Boesch and colleagues ("Altruism in Forest Chimpanzees") see more food sharing and tolerance among wild chimpanzees than has been reported in captive chimpanzees.

60. Brian Hare, "What is the Effect of Affect on Bonobo and Chimpanzee Problem Solving?" in *Neurobiology of "Umwelt": How Living Beings Perceive the World*, ed. Alain Berthoz and Yves Christen (New York: Springer, 2009), 92.

61. Richard W. Wrangham, "Ecology and Social Relationships in Two Species of Chimpanzees," in *Ecological Aspects of Social Evolution*, ed. D. Rubenstein and R. Wrangham (Princeton: Princeton University Press, 1986), 352–78.

62. Hare et al., "Tolerance Allows Bonobos to Outperform Chimpanzees on a Cooperative Task."

63. Odile Petit, Christine Desportes, and Bernard Thierry, "Differential Probability of 'Coproduction' in Two Species of Macaque (*Macaca tonkeana, M. mulatta*)," *Ethology* 90, no. 2 (1992): 107–20.

64. Hare et al., "What is the Effect of Affect on Bonobo and Chimpanzee Problem Solving?" 98.

65. Richerson and Boyd, *Not by Genes Alone*.

66. See Sarah Blaffer Hrdy, *Mothers and Others: The Evolutionary Origins of Mutual Understanding* (Cambridge, MA: Belknap Press of Harvard University Press, 2009), esp. chapter 9. See also Hrdy, *Mother Nature*.

67. Hrdy, *Mother Nature*, 247.

68. Other factors are relevant to sexual size dimorphism. Some male mammals insert a copulatory plug in the female after insemination that prevents other males from fertilizing eggs, and hence there is less intense mate competition and mate guarding, and a decrease benefit for male size—see Dunham and Rudolf, "Evolution of Sexual Size Monomorphism: The Influence of Passive Mate Guarding," *Journal of Evolutionary Biology* 22, no. 7 (2009): 1376–86. This does not seem to be a factor in human sexual behavior.

69. Randolph M. Nesse, "Runaway Social Selection for Displays of Partner Value and Altruism," *Biological Theory* 2, no. 2 (2007): 143–55.

70. Richard W. Wrangham and Dale Peterson, *Demonic Males: Apes and the Origins of Human Violence* (Boston: Houghton Mifflin, 1996).

71. Judith M. Burkart et al., "Other-Regarding Preferences in a Non-Human Primate: Common Marmosets Provision Food Altruistically," *Proceedings of the National Academy of Sciences* 104, no. 50 (2007): 19762–66.

72. Samuel Bowles, "Group Competition, Reproductive Leveling, and the Evolution of Human Altruism," *Science* 314, no. 5805 (2006): 1569–72; Jung-Kyoo Choi and Samuel Bowles, "The Coevolution of Parochial Altruism and War," *Science* 318, no. 5850 (2007): 636–40.

73. Samuel Bowles, "Did Warfare among Ancestral Hunter-Gatherers Affect the Evolution of Human Social Behaviors?" *Science* 324, no. 5932 (2009): 1293–98.

74. Nevertheless, Ernest Burch's discussion of the Iñupiaq of western Alaska (*Alliance and Conflict: The World System of the Iñupiaq Eskimos*, Lincoln: University of Nebraska Press, 2005) suggests that there was more warfare among them than early reports indicate, driven mainly by economic considerations such as competition for richer hunting territory.

5. NETWORKING

1. See Aristotle, *Nicomachean Ethics*, trans. Roger Crisp (New York: Cambridge University Press, 2000).

2. Jonathan Flint, Ralph J. Greenspan, and Kenneth S. Kendler, *How Genes Influence Behavior* (New York: Oxford University Press, 2010), 211, emphasis added.

3. R. J. Greenspan, "E Pluribus Unum, Ex Uno Plura: Quantitative and Single-Gene Perspectives on the Study of Behavior," *Annual Review of Neuroscience* 27 (2004): 79–105.

4. Ibid.

5. This is a paraphrase of Greenspan, "E Pluribus Unum," 92.

6. See Irwin Lucki, "The Spectrum of Behaviors Influenced by Serotonin," *Biological Psychiatry* 44, no. 3 (1998): 151–62. For results concerning serotonin's role in reward and negative feedback learning, see Andrea Bari et al., "Serotonin Modulates Sensitivity to Reward and Negative Feedback in a Probabilistic Reversal Learning Task in Rats," *Neuropsychopharmacology* 35, no. 6 (2010): 1290–301.

7. Klaus-Peter Lesch et al., "Association of Anxiety-Related Traits with a Polymorphism in the Serotonin Transporter Gene Regulatory Region," *Science* 274, no. 5292 (1996): 1527–31.

8. R. J. Greenspan, "The Flexible Genome," *Nature Reviews Genetics* 2, no. 5 (2001): 383–87.

9. Herman A. Dierick and Ralph J. Greenspan, "Serotonin and Neuropeptide F Have Opposite Modulatory Effects on Fly Aggression," *Nature Genetics* 39, no. 5 (2007): 678–82. Neuropeptide-F is the homologue in flies of neuropeptide-Y, linked to aggressive behavior in mammals.

10. Herman A. Dierick and Ralph J. Greenspan, "Molecular Analysis of Flies Selected for Aggressive Behavior," *Nature Genetics* 38, no. 9 (2006): 1023–31.

11. See the online supplementary material for Dierick and Greenspan, "Molecular Analysis of Flies Selected for Aggressive Behavior," table 1. It is a dramatic demonstration of the results, showing the 80 genes whose expressions were changed between the aggressive and neutral flies. Incidentally, since testosterone has often been linked to aggression, it is well worth noting that fruit flies do not have testosterone, but can be highly aggressive nonetheless.

12. Greenspan, "The Flexible Genome," "E Pluribus Unum"; and see "Genetic Networks" earlier in this chapter.

13. Dennis L. Murphy et al., "How the Serotonin Story Is Being Rewritten by New Gene-Based Discoveries Principally Related to Slc6a4, the Serotonin Transporter Gene, Which Functions to Influence All Cellular Serotonin Systems," *Neuropharmacology* 55, no. 6 (2008): 932–60.

14. Greenspan, "E Pluribus Unum," 93.

15. Flint, Greenspan, and Kendler, *How Genes Influence Behavior*. On aggression, see Larry J. Siever, "Neurobiology of Aggression and Violence," *American Journal of Psychiatry* 165, no. 4 (2008): 429–42.

16. Gleb P. Shumyatsky et al., "Identification of a Signaling Network in Lateral Nucleus of Amygdala Important for Inhibiting Memory Specifically Related to Learned Fear," *Cell* 111, no. 6 (2002): 905–18.

17. As briefly discussed in chapter 2. See also Tost et al., "A Common Allele in the Oxytocin Receptor Gene (OXTR) Impacts Prosocial Temperament."

18. Champagne and Meaney, "Like Mother, Like Daughter," "Transgenerational Effects of Social Environment."

19. Greenspan, "E Pluribus Unum," 99.

20. Jeffrey L. Elman et al., *Rethinking Innateness: A Connectionist Perspective on Development* (Cambridge, MA: MIT Press, 1996); Nicholas Evans and Stephen C. Levinson, "The Myth of Language Universals: Language Diversity and Its Importance for Cognitive Science," *Behavioral and Brain Sciences* 32, no. 5 (2009): 429–48; Morten H. Christiansen and Nick Chater, "Language as Shaped by the Brain," *Behavioral and Brain Sciences* 31, no. 5 (2008): 489–509.

21. Marc D. Hauser, *Moral Minds: How Nature Designed Our Universal Sense of Right and Wrong* (New York: Ecco, 2006).

22. Ibid., 165.

23. Ibid., xviii.

24. Flint, Greenspan, and Kendler, *How Genes Influence Behavior*.

25. On reading and genes, see Alison Gopnik, "Mind Reading," review of *Reading in the Brain—The Science and Evolution of a Human Invention*, by Stanislas Dehaene, *New York Times*, January 3, 2010.

26. See Richerson and Boyd, *Not by Genes Alone*, for a concise and compelling discussion of why the *nature versus nurture* presumption came off the rails. See also Robert C. Richardson, *Evolutionary Psychology as Maladapted Psychology* (Cambridge, MA: MIT Press, 2007).

27. Hauser, *Moral Minds*, xviii.

28. Todd Preuss, in conversation, wittily calls the "genes-for" approach "folk molecular biology," a notion I find appealing.

29. Evans and Levinson ("The Myth of Language Universals") make this point with alleged cases of linguistic universals.

30. The Inuit, who had limited access to wood, used skins for their kayaks, but if they could get driftwood, they used it for the larger whaling boats.

31. For careful criticism of claims by evolutionary psychologists, see Richardson, *Evolutionary Psychology as Maladapted Psychology*.

32. This is the fallacy of affirming the consequent (if P, then Q; Q, therefore P). One could agree that *if* a dog has fallen from 5000 feet, then it is dead. Now suppose we know that a certain dog is dead. Merely knowing that the dog is dead does not imply that it died by falling 5000 feet—maybe it died of old age, or it was run over, or it ate rat poison, and so on and on.

33. Jonathan Michael Kaplan, "Historical Evidence and Human Adaptations," *Philosophy of Science* 69, no. s3 (2002): S294–S304; David J. Buller, "Four Fallacies of Pop Evolutionary Psychology," *Scientific American* 300 (2009): 74–81.

34. Charles G. Gross, "Making Sense of Printed Symbols," *Science* 327, no. 5965 (2010): 524–25.

35. Flint, Greenspan, and Kendler, *How Genes Influence Behavior*.

36. Siever, "Neurobiology of Aggression and Violence."

37. Philip G. Zimbardo, *The Lucifer Effect: Understanding How Good People Turn Evil* (New York: Random House, 2007). Or as Stuart Anstis said in conversation, "I learned one big thing in Cambridge: never use questionnaires."

38. Bill Bryson, *At Home: A Short History of Private Life* (New York: Doubleday, 2010).

39. Graybiel, "Habits, Rituals, and the Evaluative Brain."

40. Hauser is not unaware of cultural variability on certain issues, and he is aware that intuitions can be powerful even if not innate. This makes it a little difficult to see how he designates what principles are in the innately given "moral grammar."

41. Simon Blackburn, "Response to Hauser's Tanner Lecture," unpublished, http://www.phil.cam.ac.uk/~swb24/PAPERS/Hauser.pdf.

42. Blackburn, "Response to Hauser's Tanner Lecture."

43. Christiansen and Chater, "Language as Shaped by the Brain"; Elman et al., *Rethinking Innateness*; Evans and Levinson, "The Myth of Language Universals."

44. Most of the of the papers are coauthored with Craig Joseph or with Jesse Graham; others are written solely by Haidt. For brevity, I shall refer to Haidt.

45. This list is taken from Jonathan Haidt and Jesse Graham, "Planet of the Durkheimians, Where Community, Authority, and Sacredness are Foundations of Morality," in *Social and Psychological Bases of Ideology and System Justification*, ed. J. Jost, A. C. Kay, and H. Thorisdottir (New York: Oxford University Press, 2009), 371–401. See also Jonathan Haidt and Craig Joseph, "The Moral Mind: How Five Sets of Innate Intuitions Guide the Development of Many Culture-Specific Virtues, and Perhaps Even Modules," in *The Innate Mind*, vol. 3: *Foundations and the Future*,

ed. Peter Carruthers, Stephen Laurence, and Stephen Stich (New York: Oxford University Press, 2007), 367–92; Jonathan Haidt and Craig Joseph, "Intuitive Ethics: How Innately Prepared Intuitions Generate Culturally Variable Virtues. *Daedalus* 133, no. 4 (2004): 55–66.

46. See the discussion by Flanagan, *The Really Hard Problem*, chapter 4. I have taken some liberty with the language, since the Four Noble Truths are also referred to as the Divine Abodes.

47. For a detailed and clear discussion of different lists of virtues and different ways of conceiving of fundamental virtues, see MacIntyre, *After Virtue*.

48. William J. Bennett, *The Book of Virtues: A Treasury of Great Moral Stories* (New York: Simon & Schuster, 1993).

49. For a more complete critique of Haidt's view, including his hypothesis concerning the moral differences between liberals and conservatives, see Christopher Suhler and Patricia Churchland, "Can Innate, Modular 'Foundations' Explain Morality? Challenges for Haidt's Moral Foundations Theory," *Journal of Cognitive Neuroscience* (forthcoming).

50. For a related but different critique, see Owen Flanagan and Robert Anthony Williams, "What Does the Modularity of Morals Have to Do with Ethics? Four Moral Sprouts Plus or Minus a Few," *Topics in Cognitive Science* (in press).

51. See, for example, R. Sosis and C. Alcorta, "Signaling, Solidarity, and the Sacred: The Evolution of Religious Behavior," *Evolutionary Anthropology: Issues, News, and Reviews* 12, no. 6 (2003): 264–74.

52. Michael J. Murray and Lyn Moore, "Costly Signaling and the Origin of Religion," *Journal of Cognition and Culture* 9(2009): 225–45. This article explains well what is needed by way of evidence to support an innate module hypothesis for religion.

53. Dominic Johnson, "Darwinian Selection in Asymmetric Warfare: The Natural Advantage of Insurgents and Terrorists," *Journal of the Washington Academy of Sciences* 95 (2009): 89–112.

54. David B. Larson, James P. Swyers, and Michael E. McCullough, *Scientific Research on Spirituality and Health: A Report Based on the Scientific Progress in Spirituality Conferences* (Rockville, MD: National Institute for Healthcare Research, 1998).

55. Kenneth I. Pargament et al., "Religious Struggle as a Predictor of Mortality among Medically Ill Elderly Patients: A 2-Year Longitudinal Study," *Archives of Internal Medicine* 161, no. 15 (2001): 1881–85.

56. O. Freedman et al., "Spirituality, Religion and Health: A Critical Appraisal of the Larson Reports," *Annals (Royal College of Physicians and Surgeons of Canada)* 35 (2002): 89–93.

57. William Dalrymple, *Nine Lives: In Search of the Sacred in Modern India* (London: Bloomsbury, 2009).

58. For a range of approaches, see J. Bulbulia et al., eds., *The Evolution of Religion: Studies, Theories, and Critiques* (Santa Margarita, CA: Collins Foundation Press, 2008).

59. Haidt and Graham, "Planet of the Durkheimians."

6. Skills for a Social Life

1. For an online video that shows the locations of brain structures, see http://www. youtube.com/watch?v=gVjpfPNpoGA&feature=related.

2. See Joaquin M. Fuster, *The Prefrontal Cortex* (Boston: Academic Press, 2008); A. C. Roberts, Trevor W. Robbins, and Lawrence Weiskrantz, *The Prefrontal Cortex: Executive and Cognitive Functions* (New York: Oxford University Press, 1998); David H. Zald and Scott L. Rauch, *The Orbitofrontal Cortex* (New York: Oxford University Press, 2006).

3. Todd M. Preuss, "The Cognitive Neuroscience of Human Uniqueness," in *The Cognitive Neurosciences*, ed. M. S. Gazzaniga (Cambridge, MA: MIT Press, 2009).

4. Elkhonon Goldberg and Dmitri Bougakov, "Goals, Executive Control, and Action," in *Cognition, Brain, and Consciousness: Introduction to Cognitive Neuroscience*, ed. Bernard J. Baars and Nicole M. Gage (London: Academic Press, 2007), 343.

5. Fuster, *The Prefrontal Cortex*; Josef Parvizi, "Corticocentric Myopia: Old Bias in New Cognitive Sciences," *Trends in Cognitive Sciences* 13, no. 8 (2009): 354–59.

6. For a relatively brief account, see the Siemens description, available at http://www.medical.siemens.com/siemens/de_DE/gg_mr_FBAs/files/brochures/DTI_HT_FINAL_HI.pdf.

7. Ed Bullmore and Olaf Sporns, "Complex Brain Networks: Graph Theoretical Analysis of Structural and Functional Systems," *Nature Reviews Neuroscience* 10, no. 3 (2009): 186–98; Danielle Smith Bassett and Ed Bullmore, "Small-World Brain Networks," *The Neuroscientist* 12 (2006): 512–23.

8. Elliot S. Valenstein, *Great and Desperate Cures: The Rise and Decline of Psychosurgery and Other Radical Treatments for Mental Illness* (New York: Basic Books, 1986).

9. Amy F. T. Arnsten, "Catecholamine and Second Messenger Influences on Prefrontal Cortical Networks of 'Representational Knowledge': A Rational Bridge between Genetics and the Symptoms of Mental Illness," *Cerebral Cortex* 17 (suppl. 1) (2007): 6–15; Robbins and Arnsten, "Neuropsychopharmacology of Fronto-Executive Function."

10. M. J. Crockett, "The Neurochemistry of Fairness," *Annals of the New York Academy of Sciences* 1167, no. 1 (2009): 76–86.

11. M. J. Crockett et al., "Serotonin Modulates Behavioral Reactions to Unfairness," *Science* 320, no. 5884 (2008): 1739.

12. Kaspar Meyer and Antonio Damasio, "Convergence and Divergence in a Neural Architecture for Recognition and Memory," *Trends in Neurosciences* 32, no. 7 (2009): 376–82.

13. Anne K. Churchland, Roozbeh Kiani, and Michael N. Shadlen, "Decision-Making with Multiple Alternatives." *Nature Neuroscience* 11, no. 6 (2008): 693–702.

14. I appreciate that as references to various regions with unmemorable names pile up, the eyes glaze over. For a send-up of this sort of thing by John Cleese, see http://funkwarehouse.com/jcpods/john_cleese_podcast_33.mp4.

15. Thanks to Terry Sejnowksi and his lab for the approximations.

16. For a clear account of strengths and weaknesses of fMRI, see Adina Roskies, "Neuroimaging and Inferential Distance," *Neuroethics* 1, no. 1 (2008): 19–30.

17. Leda Cosmides, John Tooby, and Jerome H. Barkow, "Introduction: Evolutionary Psychology and Conceptual Integration," in *The Adapted Mind: Evolutionary Psychology and the Generation of Culture*, ed. Jerome H. Barkow, Leda Cosmides, and John Tooby (New York: Oxford University Press, 1992), 3–15; also John Tooby and Leda Cosmides, "The Psychological Foundations of Culture," in *The Adapted Mind: Evolutionary Psychology and the Generation of Culture*, ed. J. Barkow, L. Cosmides, and J. Tooby (New York: Oxford University Press, 1992).

18. Kaspar Meyer and Antonio Damasio, "Convergence and Divergence in a Neural Architecture for Recognition and Memory," *Trends in Neurosciences* 32, no. 7 (2009): 376–82.

19. For a more detailed critique of the strong version of modularity drawing on neuroanatomy and neurophysiology, see Suhler and Churchland, "Can Innate, Modular 'Foundations' Explain Morality?" See especially section 5 on autonomous modules. On whether fMRI reveals a modular organization in the brain, see also Stephen José Hanson and Yaroslav O. Halchenko, "Brain Reading Using Full Brain Support Vector Machines for Object Recognition: There Is No 'Face' Identification Area," *Neural Computation* 20, no. 2 (2008): 486–503.

20. Russell A. Poldrack, Yaroslav O. Halchenko, and Stephen José Hanson, "Decoding the Large-Scale Structure of Brain Function by Classifying Mental States across Individuals," *Psychological Science* 20, no. 11 (2009): 1364–72.

21. Cheney and Seyfarth, *Baboon Metaphysics*, chapter 2.

22. Dunbar (*Grooming, Gossip and the Evolution of Language*) believes that we keep close track of about 150 (now known as the "Dunbar number"), but can have passing knowledge of many more.

23. Michael Tomasello, *The Cultural Origins of Human Cognition* (Cambridge, MA: Harvard University Press, 1999); Michael Tomasello et al., "Understanding and Sharing Intentions: The Origins of Cultural Cognition," *Behavioral and Brain Sciences* 28, no. 5 (2005): 675–91.

24. Albert Bandura, *Social Learning Theory* (Englewood Cliffs, NJ: Prentice Hall, 1977). See also Elizabeth Pennisi, "Conquering by Copying," *Science* 328, no. 5975 (2010): 165–67.

25. Nicky Clayton discusses this, and you can see the birds dance, at http://www .youtube.com/watch?v=y_MnwNyX0Ds.

26. Avital and Jablonka, *Animal Traditions*, 90–100.

27. Andrew Whiten, Victoria Horner, and Frans B. M. de Waal, "Conformity to Cultural Norms of Tool Use in Chimpanzees," *Nature* 437, no. 7059 (2005): 737–40; Victoria Horner and Frans B. M. de Waal, "Controlled Studies of Chimpanzee Cultural Transmission," *Progress in Brain Research* 178 (2009): 3–15. For further discussion, see also Andrew Whiten et al., "Transmission of Multiple Traditions within and between Chimpanzee Groups," *Current Biology* 17, no. 12 (2007): 1038–43; F.B.M. de Waal and K. E. Bonnie, "In Tune with Others: The Social Side of Primate Culture," in *The Question of Animal Culture*, ed. K. Laland and G. Galef (Cambridge, MA: Harvard University

Press, 2009), 19–39. For a brief but rich discussion of chimpanzee tool use, see William C. McGrew, "Chimpanzee Technology," *Science* 328, no. 5978 (2010): 579–80.

28. See S. Perry and J. H. Manson, "Traditions in Monkeys," *Evolutionary Anthropology: Issues, News, and Reviews* 12, no. 2 (2003): 71–81.

29. Pier F. Ferrari et al., "Neonatal Imitation in Rhesus Macaques," *PLoS Biology* 4, no. 9 (2006): e302.

30. Marina Davila Ross, Susanne Menzler, and Elke Zimmermann, "Rapid Facial Mimicry in Orangutan Play," *Biology Letters* 4, no. 1 (2008): 27–30.

31. Panksepp, *Affective Neuroscience*, chapter 15.

32. Steven Quartz and Terrence J. Sejnowski, *Liars, Lovers, and Heroes: What the New Brain Science Reveals About How We Become Who We Are* (New York: William Morrow, 2002), chapter 2.

33. Jay A. Gottfried, John O'Doherty, and Raymond J. Dolan, "Encoding Predictive Reward Value in Human Amygdala and Orbitofrontal Cortex," *Science* 301, no. 5636 (2003): 1104–7; Ann M. Graybiel, "The Basal Ganglia: Learning New Tricks and Loving It," *Current Opinion in Neurobiology* 15, no. 6 (2005): 638–44.

34. R. M. Hare, *Moral Thinking: Its Levels, Method, and Point* (Oxford: Clarendon Press, 1981).

35. Blackburn, "Response to Hauser's Tanner Lecture."

36. For the conditions motivating change, see Boyd and Richerson, "Solving the Puzzle of Human Cooperation."

37. Hickok, "Eight Problems." See also Gregory Hickok, Kayoko Okada, and John T. Serences, "Area SPT in the Human Planum Temporale Supports Sensory-Motor Integration for Speech Processing," *Journal of Neurophysiology* 101, no. 5 (2009): 2725–32.

38. Nathan J. Emery and Nicola S. Clayton, "Comparative Social Cognition," *Annual Review of Psychology* 60, no. 1 (2008): 87–113; Clayton, Dally, and Emery, "Social Cognition by Food-Caching Corvids."

39. Following Chris D. Frith and Uta Frith, "The Neural Basis of Mentalizing," *Neuron* 50, no. 4 (2006): 531–34.

40. Vittorio Gallese, "Motor Abstraction: A Neuroscientific Account of How Action Goals and Intentions Are Mapped and Understood," *Psychological Research* 73, no. 4 (2009): 486–98; Giacomo Rizzolatti and Laila Craighero, "The Mirror-Neuron System," *Annual Review of Neuroscience* 27, no. 1 (2004): 169–92.

41. G. Pellegrino et al., "Understanding Motor Events: A Neurophysiological Study," *Experimental Brain Research* 91, no. 1 (1992): 176–80. For a review of the history, see Giacomo Rizzolatti and Maddalena Fabbri-Destro, "Mirror Neurons: From Discovery to Autism," *Experimental Brain Research* 200, no. 3 (2010): 223–37.

42. Vittorio Gallese et al., "Action Recognition in the Premotor Cortex," *Brain* 119, no. 2 (1996): 593–609.

43. Leonardo Fogassi et al., "Parietal Lobe: From Action Organization to Intention Understanding," *Science* 308, no. 5722 (2005): 662–67.

44. Gallese, "Motor Abstraction"; Lindsay M. Oberman et al., "EEG Evidence for Mirror Neuron Dysfunction in Autism Spectrum Disorders," *Cognitive Brain Research* 24, no. 2 (2005): 190–98.

45. Vittorio Gallese and Alvin Goldman, "Mirror Neurons and the Simulation Theory of Mind-Reading," *Trends in Cognitive Sciences* 2, no. 12 (1998): 493–501. For detailed criticism of this claim, see Rebecca Saxe, "The Neural Evidence for Simulation Is Weaker Than I Think You Think It Is," *Philosophical Studies* 144, no. 3 (2009): 447–56.

46. Fogassi et al., "Parietal Lobe," 665.

47. Cecilia Heyes, "Where Do Mirror Neurons Come From?" *Neuroscience & Biobehavioral Reviews* 34, no. 4 (2010): 575–83. Meyer and Damasio, "Convergence and Divergence in a Neural Architecture for Recognition and Memory."

48. See the discussion by Erhan Oztop, Mitsuo Kawato, and Michael Arbib, "Mirror Neurons and Imitation: A Computationally Guided Review," *Neural Networks* 19, no. 3 (2006): 254–71. For criticism of the simulation-mirror neuron story, see Pierre Jacob, "What Do Mirror Neurons Contribute to Human Social Cognition?" *Mind & Language* 23, no. 2 (2008): 190–223. See also Gregory Hickok, "Eight Problems for the Mirror Neuron Theory of Action Understanding in Monkeys and Humans," *Journal of Cognitive Neuroscience* 21, no. 7 (2009): 1229–43.

49. Fogassi et al., "Parietal Lobe," 666. See also Marco Iacoboni et al., "Grasping the Intentions of Others with One's Own Mirror Neuron System," *PLoS Biology* 3, no. 3 (2005): e79.

50. Hickok, "Eight Problems."

51. Oztop, Kawato, and Arbib, "Mirror Neurons and Imitation."

52. Pierre Jacob and Marc Jeannerod ("The Motor Theory of Social Cognition: A Critique," *Trends in Cognitive Sciences* 9, no. 1 [2005]: 21–25) make this point regarding mirror neuron hypotheses in general.

53. In fairness, I should note that Oztop, Kawato, and Arbib are not claiming to explain mental attribution in general, and are clear about the limitations of their model.

54. Marc A. Sommer and Robert H. Wurtz, "Brain Circuits for the Internal Monitoring of Movements," *Annual Review of Neuroscience* 31, no. 1 (2008): 317–38.

55. See also Robert P. Spunt, Ajay B. Satpute, and Matthew D. Lieberman, "Identifying the What, Why, and How of an Observed Action: An fMRI Study of Mentalizing and Mechanizing During Action Observation," *Journal of Cognitive Neuroscience* (2010): 1–12; Scott T. Grafton and Antonia F. de C. Hamilton, "Evidence for a Distributed Hierarchy of Action Representation in the Brain," *Human Movement Science* 26, no. 4 (2007): 590–616; Susan S. Jones, "Imitation in Infancy," *Psychological Science* 18, no. 7 (2007): 593–99.

56. For discussion of this and related phenomena, see Matthew Roser and Michael S. Gazzaniga, "Automatic Brains—Interpretive Minds," *Current Directions in Psychological Science* 13, no. 2 (2004): 56–59.

57. Richard E. Nisbett and Timothy D. Wilson, "Telling More Than We Can Know: Verbal Reports on Mental Processes," *Psychological Review* 8 (1977): 231–59.

58. Petter Johansson et al., "Failure to Detect Mismatches between Intention and Outcome in a Simple Decision Task," *Science* 310, no. 5745 (2005): 116–19.

59. See a surprising discussion of reasoning by Hugo Mercier and Dan Sperber, "Why Do Humans Reason? Arguments for an Argumentative Theory," *Behavioral and Brain Sciences* (in press).

60. Tucker, Luu, and Derryberry, "Love Hurts"; G. Buzsáki, *Rhythms of the Brain* (Oxford: Oxford University Press, 2006).

61. Roy F. Baumeister and E. J. Masicampo, "Conscious Thought Is for Facilitating Social and Cultural Interactions: How Mental Simulations Serve the Animal-Culture Interface," *Psychological Review* 117, no. 3 (2010): 945–71.

62. Though see, in the following section, the discussion of data on pain during surgery from W. D. Hutchison et al. ("Pain-Related Neurons in the Human Cingulate Cortex," *Nature Neuroscience* 2, no. 5 [1999]: 403–5).

63. For discussion of group versus single-subject analyses, see India Morrison and Paul E. Downing, "Organization of Felt and Seen Pain Responses in Anterior Cingulate Cortex," *Neuroimage* 37, no. 2 (2007): 642–51.

64. Valeria Gazzola and Christian Keysers, "The Observation and Execution of Actions Share Motor and Somatosensory Voxels in All Tested Subjects: Single-Subject Analyses of Unsmoothed fMRI Data," *Cerebral Cortex* 19, no. 6 (2009): 1239–55.

65. See Hickok, "Eight Problems." Studies of human patients with brain damage give rather mixed answers, and as Hickok notes, patients with damage confined to Broca's area do not seem to have deficits in language comprehension or in attributing intentions and goals.

66. See also Spunt, Satpute, and Lieberman, "Identifying the What, Why, and How of an Observed Action"; Grafton and Hamilton, "Evidence for a Distributed Hierarchy of Action Representation."

67. Liane Young and Rebecca Saxe, "An fMRI Investigation of Spontaneous Mental State Inference for Moral Judgment," *Journal of Cognitive Neuroscience* 21, no. 7 (2008): 1396–405. See also Frith and Frith, "The Neural Basis of Mentalizing."

68. John-Dylan Haynes et al., "Reading Hidden Intentions in the Human Brain," *Current Biology* 17, no. 4 (2007): 323–28. See also Todd S. Braver and Susan R. Bongiolatti, "The Role of Frontopolar Cortex in Subgoal Processing During Working Memory," *Neuroimage* 15, no. 3 (2002): 523–36.

69. See Alvin Goldman and Frederique de Vignemont, "Is Social Cognition Embodied?" *Trends in Cognitive Sciences* 13, no. 4 (2009): 154–59.

70. Marco Iacoboni, "Neurobiology of Imitation," *Current Opinion in Neurobiology* 19, no. 6 (2009): 663.

71. See Marco Iacoboni, *Mirroring People: The New Science of How We Connect with Others* (New York: Farrar, Straus and Giroux, 2008), 111 ff.

72. Bruno Wicker et al., "Both of Us Disgusted in My Insula: The Common Neural Basis of Seeing and Feeling Disgust," *Neuron* 40, no. 3 (2003): 655–64.

73. Hutchison et al., "Pain-Related Neurons in the Human Cingulate Cortex."

74. Grit Hein and Tania Singer, "I Feel How You Feel but Not Always: The Empathic Brain and Its Modulation," *Current Opinion in Neurobiology* 18, no. 2 (2008): 153–58. See also the following two reviews: J.A.C.J. Bastiaansen, M. Thioux, and C. Keysers, "Evidence for Mirror Systems in Emotions," *Philosophical Transactions of the Royal Society B: Biological Sciences* 364, no. 1528 (2009): 2391–404; Christian Keysers, Jon H. Kaas, and Valeria Gazzola, "Somatosensation in Social Perception," *Nature Reviews Neuroscience* 11, no. 6 (2010): 417–28.

75. Yawei Cheng et al., "Expertise Modulates the Perception of Pain in Others," *Current Biology* 17, no. 19 (2007): 1708–13.

76. Cheng et al., "Love Hurts: An fMRI Study."

77. Barbara Wild et al., "Why Are Smiles Contagious? An fMRI Study of the Interaction between Perception of Facial Affect and Facial Movements," *Psychiatry Research* 123, no. 1 (2003): 17–36.

78. Lindsay M. Oberman, Piotr Winkielman, and Vilayanur S. Ramachandran, "Face to Face: Blocking Facial Mimicry Can Selectively Impair Recognition of Emotional Expressions," *Social Neuroscience* 2, no. 3–4 (2007): 167–78.

79. Morrison and Downing, "Organization of Felt and Seen Pain Responses in Anterior Cingulate Cortex."

80. Iacoboni, *Mirroring People*, "Neurobiology of Imitation."

81. See Mbemba Jabbi and Christian Keysers, "Inferior Frontal Gyrus Activity Triggers Anterior Insula Response to Emotional Facial Expressions," *Emotion* 8 (2008): 775–80, for a report addressing causality.

82. Ralph Adolphs et al., "A Mechanism for Impaired Fear Recognition after Amygdala Damage," *Nature* 433, no. 7021 (2005): 68–72; Adam K. Anderson and Elizabeth A. Phelps, "Is the Human Amygdala Critical for the Subjective Experience of Emotion? Evidence of Intact Dispositional Affect in Patients with Amygdala Lesions," *Journal of Cognitive Neuroscience* 14, no. 5 (2006): 709–20; Christian Keysers and Valeria Gazzola, "Towards a Unifying Neural Theory of Social Cognition," *Progress in Brain Research* 156 (2006): 379–401. Perhaps, as Bastiaansen and colleagues ("Evidence for Mirror Systems in Emotions") suggest, the amygdala is only indirectly supporting fear processing, and may be primarily connected to attentional processes.

83. Elizabeth A. Ascher et al., "Relationship Satisfaction and Emotional Language in Frontotemporal Dementia and Alzheimer Disease Patients and Spousal Caregivers," *Alzheimer Disease & Associated Disorders* 24, no. 1 (2010): 49–55.

84. S.-J. Blakemore et al., "Somatosensory Activations During the Observation of Touch and a Case of Vision-Touch Synaesthesia," *Brain* 128, no. 7 (2005): 1571–83.

85. Alvin I. Goldman, *Simulating Minds: The Philosophy, Psychology, and Neuroscience of Mindreading* (New York: Oxford University Press, 2006).

86. Stephanie D. Preston and Frans B. M. de Waal, "Empathy: Its Ultimate and Proximate Bases," *Behavioral and Brain Sciences* 25, no. 1 (2001): 1–20.

87. Cheng et al., "Love Hurts: An fMRI Study."

88. A. N. Meltzoff, "Roots of Social Cognition: The Like-Me Framework," in *Minnesota Symposia on Child Psychology: Meeting the Challenge of Translational Research in Child Psychology*, ed. D. Cicchetti and M. R. Gunnar (Hoboken, NJ: Wiley, 2009), 29–58.

89. Buzsáki, *Rhythms of the Brain*, 371.

90. Iacoboni, "Neurobiology of Imitation."

91. Pascal Molenberghs, Ross Cunnington, and Jason B. Mattingley, "Is the Mirror Neuron System Involved in Imitation? A Short Review and Meta-Analysis," *Neuroscience & Biobehavioral Reviews* 33, no. 7 (2009): 975–80.

92. Susan S. Jones, "The Role of Mirror Neurons in Imitation: A Commentary on Gallese," in *Perspectives on Imitation: From Neuroscience to Social Science*, vol. 1: *Mechanisms of Imitation and Imitation in Animals*, ed. Susan Hurley and Nick Chater (Cambridge, MA: MIT Press, 2005), 205–10.

93. Simon Baron-Cohen, *Mindblindness: An Essay on Autism and Theory of Mind* (Cambridge, MA: MIT Press, 1995).

94. Justin Williams, Andrew Whiten, and Tulika Singh, "A Systematic Review of Action Imitation in Autistic Spectrum Disorder," *Journal of Autism and Developmental Disorders* 34, no. 3 (2004): 285–99.

95. John R. Hughes, "Update on Autism: A Review of 1300 Reports Published in 2008," *Epilepsy & Behavior* 16, no. 4 (2009): 569–89.

96. See Sally Ozonoff, Bruce F. Pennington, and Sally J. Rogers, "Executive Function Deficits in High-Functioning Autistic Individuals: Relationship to Theory of Mind," *Journal of Child Psychology and Psychiatry* 32, no. 7 (1991): 1081–105.

97. Daniel N. McIntosh et al., "When the Social Mirror Breaks: Deficits in Automatic, but Not Voluntary, Mimicry of Emotional Facial Expressions in Autism," *Developmental Science* 9, no. 3 (2006): 295–302.

98. Oberman, Winkielman, and Ramachandran, "Face to Face."

99. M. Dapretto et al., "Understanding Emotions in Others: Mirror Neuron Dysfunction in Children with Autism Spectrum Disorders," *Nature Neuroscience* 9, no. 1 (2006): 28–30.

100. Lindsay M. Oberman, Jaime A. Pineda, and Vilayanur S. Ramachandran, "The Human Mirror Neuron System: A Link between Action Observation and Social Skills," *Social Cognitive and Affective Neuroscience* 2, no. 1 (2007): 62–66.

101. Ruth Raymaekers, Jan Roelf Wiersema, and Herbert Roeyers, "EEG Study of the Mirror Neuron System in Children with High Functioning Autism," *Brain Research* 1304 (2009): 113–21.

102. Claudio Tennie, Josep Call, and Michael Tomasello, "Ratcheting up the Ratchet: On the Evolution of Cumulative Culture," *Philosophical Transactions of the Royal Society B: Biological Sciences* 364, no. 1528 (2009): 2405–15.

103. T. L. Chartrand and J. A. Bargh, "The Chameleon Effect: The Perception-Behavior Link and Social Interaction," *Journal of Personality and Social Psychology* 76, no. 6 (1999): 893–910; Clara Michelle Cheng and Tanya L. Chartrand, "Self-Monitoring without Awareness: Using Mimicry as a Nonconscious Affiliation Strategy," *Journal of Personality and Social Psychology* 85, no. 6 (2003): 1170–79; J. L. Lakin and T. L. Chartrand, "Using Nonconscious Behavioral Mimicry to Create Affiliation and Rapport," *Psychological Science* 14, no. 4 (2003): 334–39; Jessica L. Lakin et al., "The Chameleon Effect as Social Glue: Evidence for the Evolutionary Significance of Nonconscious Mimicry," *Journal of Nonverbal Behavior* 27, no. 3 (2003): 145–62.

104. See Lakin et al., "The Chameleon Effect as Social Glue."

105. Chris D. Frith, "Social Cognition," *Philosophical Transactions of the Royal Society B: Biological Sciences* 363, no. 1499 (2008): 2033–39; Tomasello et al., "Understanding and Sharing Intentions."

106. Hrdy, *Mother Nature*.

107. Masako Myowa-Yamakoshi et al., "Imitation in Neonatal Chimpanzees (*Pan troglodytes*)," *Developmental Science* 7, no. 4 (2004): 437–42; Ferrari et al., "Neonatal Imitation in Rhesus Macaques"; Davila Ross, Menzler, and Zimmermann, "Rapid Facial Mimicry in Orangutan Play."

108. Susan S. Jones, "Infants Learn to Imitate by Being Imitated," in *Proceedings of the International Conference on Development and Learning (ICDL)*, ed. C. Yu, L. B. Smith, and O. Sporns (Bloomington: Indiana University, 2006).

109. When I was a graduate student in Oxford, I was expected to attend the regular sherry parties that my tutor at Balliol College held for his male undergraduates. I was always uncomfortable, because as a colonial, and a country bumpkin to boot, I did not have the slightest idea how I should behave. Trying to assimilate the ways of young Englishmen educated at British "public" (private) schools was, quite simply, beyond me. Needless to say, with the exception of a very awkward Irish lad who was comparably handicapped socially, no one ever talked to me for more than a minute.

110. Liam Kavanagh et al., "People who mimic unfriendly individuals suffer reputational costs" (submitted).

111. Richerson and Boyd, *Not by Genes Alone*.

7. Not as a Rule

1. Peter J. Bayley, Jennifer C. Frascino, and Larry R. Squire, "Robust Habit Learning in the Absence of Awareness and Independent of the Medial Temporal Lobe," *Nature* 436, no. 7050 (2005): 550–53; Aaron R. Seitz et al., "Unattended Exposure to Components of Speech Sounds Yields Same Benefits as Explicit Auditory Training," *Cognition* 115, no. 3 (2010): 435–43.

2. Across cultures, the threshold for helping without insult varies. The Inuit generally have a higher threshold for when help can be offered to an adult without insult, and to the naïve, this can be misunderstood as indifference to one's struggle righting a kayak, for example.

3. For a less momentous example, see the article by Edward C. Wallace, "Putting Vendors in Their Place" (*New York Times*, April 17, 2010), regarding unregulated vendors of "written material" in public spaces in New York.

4. Johnson, *Moral Imagination*.

5. A. C. Grayling, *What Is Good? The Search for the Best Way to Live* (London: Weidenfeld & Nicolson, 2003), 9–55.

6. Michael S. Bendiksby and Michael L. Platt, "Neural Correlates of Reward and Attention in Macaque Area LIP," *Neuropsychologia* 44, no. 12 (2006): 2411–20; Anne K. Churchland, Roozbeh Kiani, and Michael N. Shadlen, "Decision-Making with Multiple Alternatives," *Nature Neuroscience* 11, no. 6 (2008): 693–702; Robert O. Deaner, Stephen V. Shepherd, and Michael L. Platt, "Familiarity Accentuates Gaze Cuing in Women but Not Men," *Biology Letters* 3, no. 1 (2007): 65–68.

7. Graybiel, "Habits, Rituals, and the Evaluative Brain."

8. Suhler and Churchland, "Control: Conscious and Otherwise."

9. Robert C. Solomon, *Introducing Philosophy: A Text with Integrated Readings* (New York: Oxford University Press, 2008), 487.

10. See, e.g., John Rawls, *A Theory of Justice* (Oxford: Clarendon Press, 1972).

11. Flanagan, *The Really Hard Problem*, 140.

12. Johnson, *Moral Imagination*, 5.

13. Simon Blackburn, *Ethics: A Very Short Introduction* (New York: Oxford University Press, 2003).

14. Marc Bekoff, *Animal Passions and Beastly Virtues: Reflections on Redecorating Nature* (Philadelphia: Temple University Press, 2006). Bekoff and Pierce, *Wild Justice*; Boesch et al., "Altruism in Forest Chimpanzees."

15. Souter, David. "Commencement Address to Harvard University." http://news .harvard.edu/gazette/story/2010/05/text-of-justice-david-souters-speech/, Spring 2010.

16. Edward Slingerland, "Toward an Empirically Responsible Ethics: Cognitive Science, Virtue Ethics and Effortless Attention in Early Chinese Thought," in *Effortless Attention: A New Perspective in the Cognitive Science of Attention and Action*, ed. Brian Bruya (Cambridge, MA: MIT Press, 2010), 247–86.

17. See Sheri Fink, "The Deadly Choices at Memorial," *New York Times Magazine*, August 30, 2009.

18. Stephen Anderson, "The Golden Rule: Not So Golden Anymore," *Philosophy Now*, July/August 2009.

19. Both vaccinations and anesthetics were vigorously opposed by Christians who saw them as interfering with the work of God. See Patricia S. Churchland, "Human Dignity from a Neurophilosophical Perspective," in *Human Dignity and Bioethics: Essays Commissioned by the President's Council on Bioethics* (Washington, DC: President's Council on Bioethics, 2008), 99–121.

20. La Cerra and Bingham, *The Origin of Minds*, chapters 3 and 4.

21. Blackburn, *How to Read Hume*.

22. Here is the categorical imperative itself, in Kant's words (as translated by Mary Gregor): "act only in accordance with that maxim through which you can at the same time will that it become a universal law" (Kant, *Groundwork of the Metaphysics of Morals*, New York: Cambridge University Press, 1998). In an accessible discussion, Robert Johnson ("Kant's Moral Philosophy," in *The Stanford Encyclopedia of Philosophy* [Winter 2009 Edition], ed. Edward N. Zalta, 2008, http://plato.stanford.edu/ archives/win2009/entries/kant-moral) explains the decision procedure as follows:

> First, formulate a maxim that enshrines your reason for acting as you propose. Second, recast that maxim as a universal law of nature governing all rational agents, and so as holding that all must, by natural law, act as you yourself propose to act in these circumstances. Third, consider whether your maxim is even conceivable in a world governed by this law of nature. If it is, then, fourth, ask yourself whether you would, or could, rationally *will* to act on your maxim in such a world. If you could, then your action is morally permissible.

As an undergraduate exposed to this idea, I had to suspect that kind and virtuous people in fact rarely, if ever, go through this procedure—or even that we would *want* them to.

23. See also Blackburn, *Ethics: A Very Short Introduction*.

24. Ronald De Sousa, *The Rationality of Emotion* (Cambridge, MA: MIT Press, 1987); Ronald De Sousa, *Why Think? Evolution and the Rational Mind* (New York: Oxford University Press, 2007); Flanagan, *The Really Hard Problem*; Johnson, *Moral Imagination*.

25. For a detailed discussion of the texts, see D. G. Brown, "Mill's Moral Theory: Ongoing Revisionism," *Politics, Philosophy, & Economics* 9, no. 1 (2010): 5–45.

26. See Dale Jamieson, "When Utilitarians Should Be Virtue Theorists," *Utilitas* 19, no. 2 (2007): 160–83.

27. John Stuart Mill, *Utilitarianism*, in *On Liberty and Other Essays*, ed. John Gray (New York: Oxford University Press, 1998), 129–201. Mill scholarship is both voluminous and complicated, so the brief discussion here is necessarily just a sketch.

28. See again Justice Souter's commencement address to Harvard University.

29. As, for example, Richard Dawkins and Christopher Hitchens propose for the Pope's visit to England. This makes many Roman Catholics unhappy, possibly very unhappy, but we allow it even so.

30. Brown, "Mill's Moral Theory."

31. Ibid., 16.

32. See, for instance, Peter Singer, *Animal Liberation: A New Ethics for Our Treatment of Animals* (New York: Random House, 1975), and *Practical Ethics* (New York: Cambridge University Press, 1979).

33. See Singer's discussion in the edited volume *Peter Singer under Fire: The Moral Iconoclast Faces His Critics*, ed. Jeffrey Schaler (Chicago: Open Court, 2009), esp. pp. 421–24. See also Thomas Nagel, "What Peter Singer Wants of You," *New York Review of Books*, March 25, 2010.

34. Thomas Scanlon, *The Difficulty of Tolerance: Essays in Political Philosophy* (New York: Cambridge University Press, 2003), 131 (my italics).

35. Most day-to-day categories have radial structure, with prototypes at the center, and other examples of lesser degrees of similarity radiating out from the center. That moral categories are similarly organized—prototypes at the center where agreement is strong, intermediate cases that are less clear cut, and fuzzy boundaries where disagreements abound—explains a lot of human discussion and moral negotiation. It is also consistent with the observation that the disagreements of moral philosophers, as well as of most others, are not about the prototypical cases, but the cases at a similarity distance from the prototypes. Some of the debates among academic consequentialists are the moral equivalent of disagreeing about whether parsley is a vegetable, not about whether carrots are a vegetable. Others, however, are important and painfully unresolved, such as disagreements about making organ donation the default case or allowing parents to withhold medical treatment from children on religious grounds.

36. William D. Casebeer, *Natural Ethical Facts: Evolution, Connectionism, and Moral Cognition* (Cambridge, MA: MIT Press, 2003); Sam Harris, *The Moral Landscape: How Science Can Determine Human Values* (New York: Free Press, 2010).

37. Flanagan, *The Really Hard Problem*, 141.

38. Paul M. Churchland, "Toward a Cognitive Neurobiology of the Moral Virtues," *Topoi* 17 (1998): 1–14.

39. Steven Bogaerts and David Leake, "A Framework for Rapid and Modular Case-Based Reasoning System Development," Technical Report TR 617, Computer Science Department, Indiana University, Bloomington, IN, 2005; Jonathan Haidt, "The Emotional Dog and Its Rational Tail: A Social Intuitionist Approach to Moral Judgment," *Psychological Review* 108, no. 4 (2001): 814–34; David B. Leake, *Case-Based Reasoning: Experiences, Lessons and Future Directions* (Cambridge, MA: MIT Press, 1996).

40. See the essays in Dedre Gentner, Keith James Holyoak, and Boicho N. Kokinov's collection *The Analogical Mind: Perspectives from Cognitive Science* (Cambridge, MA: MIT Press, 2001).

41. See Churchland, "Inference to the Best Decision."

42. Paul M. Churchland, "Rules, Know-How, and the Future of Moral Cognition," in *Moral Epistemology Naturalized*, ed. Richmond Campbell and Bruce Hunter (Calgary: University of Calgary Press, 2000), 291–306; George Lakoff and Mark Johnson, *Philosophy in the Flesh: The Embodied Mind and Its Challenge to Western Thought* (New York: Basic Books, 1999); Johnson, *Moral Imagination*.

43. Bernard Gert, "The Definition of Morality," in *The Stanford Encyclopedia of Philosophy* (Fall 2008 edition), ed. Edward N. Zalta, 2008, http://plato.stanford.edu/entries/morality-definition/, emphasis added.

44. Notable exceptions include Mark Johnson, A. C. Grayling, William Casebeer, Owen Flanagan, Simon Blackburn, Neil Levy, and Alasdair McIntyre.

45. G. E. Moore, *Principia Ethica* (Cambridge: Cambridge University Press, 1903). For approving comments concerning the naturalistic fallacy, see, for example, Joshua Greene, "From Neural 'Is' to Moral 'Ought': What Are the Moral Implications of Neuroscientific Moral Psychology?" *Nature Reviews Neuroscience* 4, no. 10 (2003): 847–50.

46. See the very clear discussion of Moore by Thomas Hurka, "Moore's Moral Philosophy" in the *Stanford Encyclopedia of Philosophy*, ed. Edward M. Zalta, January 2005, with revisions in March 2010, http://plato.stanford.edu/entries/moore-moral/.

47. Grayling, *What Is Good?* chapter 8.

8. Religion and Morality

1. Francis S. Collins, *The Language of God: A Scientist Presents Evidence for Belief* (New York: Free Press, 2006).

2. I am not suggesting I enjoyed wringing their necks, but I did overcome reticence about it, and if it is done quickly, the hen does not suffer.

3. Franklin Graham, *The Name* (Nashville, TN: Thomas Nelson Publishers, 2002).

4. Socrates actually uses the word "piety," but meant by that word what we mean by *good*.

5. For an updated view of this, see William Casebeer's *Natural Ethical Facts*, and Owen Flanagan's *Varieties of Moral Personality: Ethics and Psychological Realism* (Cambridge, MA: Harvard University Press, 1991).

6. The full text of Leviticus 25:44–46 (King James version) reads as follows:

[44] Both thy bondmen, and thy bondmaids, which thou shalt have, shall be of the heathen that are round about you; of them shall ye buy bondmen and bondmaids.

[45] Moreover of the children of the strangers that do sojourn among you, of them shall ye buy, and of their families that are with you, which they begat in your land: and they shall be your possession.

[46] And ye shall take them as an inheritance for your children after you, to inherit them for a possession; they shall be your bondmen for ever: but over your brethren the children of Israel, ye shall not rule one over another with rigour.

7. For a more complete discussion of this problem, see earlier, chapter 7, on rules.

8. For example, this Confucian caution: "He who would take revenge should dig two graves."

9. And biological—see Pascal Boyer, *Religion Explained: The Evolutionary Origins of Religious Thought* (New York: Basic Books, 2001), and Loyal D. Rue, *Religion Is Not About God: How Spiritual Traditions Nurture Our Biological Nature and What to Expect When They Fail* (New Brunswick, NJ: Rutgers University Press, 2005).

10. See Flanagan's witty but also serious discussion in chapter 6 of *The Really Hard Problem*.

11. Collins's remarks, which come from a lecture given at UC-Berkeley in 2008, are recounted and discussed in Sam Harris, "Science Is in the Details," *New York Times*, July 26, 2009.

12. Although this remark is commonly attributed to Fyodor Dostoevsky, the most that can be said is that something along those lines is espoused by the character Ivan Karamazov in Dostoevsky's novel, *The Brothers Karamazov*. There is some suggestion that the remark was made by Sartre in discussing *The Brothers Karamazov*, though this obviously does not imply that Sartre himself believed it.

13. See also Harris, *The Moral Landscape*.

14. Blackburn, *How to Read Hume*.

15. The data bear this out—see Henrich et al., "Markets, Religion, Community Size, and the Evolution of Fairness and Punishment."

16. For a recent, deep discussion of these issues, see Douglass C. North, John Joseph Wallis, and Barry R. Weingast, *Violence and Social Orders: A Conceptual Framework for Interpreting Recorded Human History* (Cambridge: Cambridge University Press, 2009).

Bibliography

Adolphs, Ralph, Frederic Gosselin, Tony W. Buchanan, Daniel Tranel, Philippe Schyns, and Antonio R. Damasio. "A Mechanism for Impaired Fear Recognition after Amygdala Damage." *Nature* 433, no. 7021 (2005): 68–72.

Andari, Elissar, Jean-René Duhamel, Tiziana Zalla, Evelyn Herbrecht, Marion Leboyer, and Angela Sirigu. "Promoting Social Behavior with Oxytocin in High-Functioning Autism Spectrum Disorders." *Proceedings of the National Academy of Sciences* 107, no. 9 (2010): 4389–94.

Anderson, Adam K., and Elizabeth A. Phelps. "Is the Human Amygdala Critical for the Subjective Experience of Emotion? Evidence of Intact Dispositional Affect in Patients with Amygdala Lesions." *Journal of Cognitive Neuroscience* 14, no. 5 (2006): 709–20.

Anderson, Stephen. "The Golden Rule: Not So Golden Anymore." *Philosophy Now*, July/August 2009.

Aristotle. *Nicomachean Ethics*. Translated by Roger Crisp. New York: Cambridge University Press, 2000.

Arnsten, Amy F. T. "Catecholamine and Second Messenger Influences on Prefrontal Cortical Networks of "Representational Knowledge": A Rational Bridge between Genetics and the Symptoms of Mental Illness." *Cerebral Cortex* 17 (2007): 6–15.

Ascher, Elizabeth A., Virginia E. Sturm, Benjamin H. Seider, Sarah R. Holley, Bruce L. Miller, and Robert W. Levenson. "Relationship Satisfaction and Emotional Language in Frontotemporal Dementia and Alzheimer Disease Patients and Spousal Caregivers." *Alzheimer Disease & Associated Disorders* 24, no. 1 (2010): 49–55.

Avital, Eytan, and Eva Jablonka. *Animal Traditions: Behavioural Inheritance in Evolution*. New York: Cambridge University Press, 2000.

Baier, Annette. *A Progress of Sentiments: Reflections on Hume's Treatise*. Cambridge, MA: Harvard University Press, 1991.

Bales, Karen L., Albert J. Kim, Antoniah D. Lewis-Reese, and C. Sue Carter. "Both Oxytocin and Vasopressin May Influence Alloparental Behavior in Male Prairie Voles." *Hormones and Behavior* 45, no. 5 (2004): 354–61.

Bales, Karen L., Kristin M. Kramer, Antoniah D. Lewis-Reese, and C. Sue Carter. "Effects of Stress on Parental Care Are Sexually Dimorphic in Prairie Voles." *Physiology & Behavior* 87, no. 2 (2006): 424–29.

Bales, Karen L., P. M. Plotsky, L. J. Young, M. M. Lim, N. Grotte, E. Ferrer, and C. S. Carter. "Neonatal Oxytocin Manipulations Have Long-Lasting, Sexually Dimorphic Effects on Vasopressin Receptors." *Neuroscience* 144, no. 1 (2007): 38–45.

Bales, Karen L., Julie A. van Westerhuyzen, Antoniah D. Lewis-Reese, Nathaniel D. Grotte, Jalene A. Lanter, and C. Sue Carter. "Oxytocin Has Dose-Dependent Developmental Effects on Pair-Bonding and Alloparental Care in Female Prairie Voles." *Hormones and Behavior* 52, no. 2 (2007): 274–79.

Bandura, Albert. *Social Learning Theory*. Englewood Cliffs, NJ: Prentice Hall, 1977.

Bari, Andrea, David E. Theobald, Daniele Caprioli, Adam C. Mar, Alex Aidoo-Micah, Jeffrey W. Dalley, and Trevor W. Robbins. "Serotonin Modulates Sensitivity to Reward and Negative Feedback in a Probabilistic Reversal Learning Task in Rats." *Neuropsychopharmacology* 35, no. 6 (2010): 1290–301.

Baron-Cohen, Simon. *Mindblindness: An Essay on Autism and Theory of Mind*, Learning, Development, and Conceptual Change. Cambridge, MA: MIT Press, 1995.

Bassett, Danielle Smith, and Ed Bullmore. "Small-World Brain Networks." *The Neuroscientist* 12 (2006): 512–523.

Bastiaansen, J. A. C. J., M. Thioux, and C. Keysers. "Evidence for Mirror Systems in Emotions." *Philosophical Transactions of the Royal Society B: Biological Sciences* 364, no. 1528 (2009): 2391–404.

Baumeister, Roy F. *The Cultural Animal: Human Nature, Meaning, and Social Life*. New York: Oxford University Press, 2005.

Baumeister, Roy F., and Eli J. Finkel, eds. *Advanced Social Psychology: The State of the Science*. New York: Oxford University Press, 2010.

Baumeister, Roy F., and E. J. Masicampo. "Conscious Thought Is for Facilitating Social and Cultural Interactions: How Mental Simulations Serve the Animal-Culture Interface." *Psychological Review* 117, no. 3 (2010): 945–71.

Baumgartner, Thomas, Markus Heinrichs, Aline Vonlanthen, Urs Fischbacher, and Ernst Fehr. "Oxytocin Shapes the Neural Circuitry of Trust and Trust Adaptation in Humans." *Neuron* 58, no. 4 (2008): 639–50.

Bayley, Peter J., Jennifer C. Frascino, and Larry R. Squire. "Robust Habit Learning in the Absence of Awareness and Independent of the Medial Temporal Lobe." *Nature* 436, no. 7050 (2005): 550–53.

Bekoff, Marc. *Animal Passions and Beastly Virtues: Reflections on Redecorating Nature*. Philadelphia: Temple University Press, 2006.

Bekoff, Marc, and Jessica Pierce. *Wild Justice: The Moral Lives of Animals*. Chicago: University of Chicago Press, 2009.

Belkin, Lisa. "The Evolution of Dad," *New York Times Magazine*, June 16, 2010; http://parenting.blogs.nytimes.com/2010/06/16/the-evolution-of-dad/.

Bendiksby, Michael S., and Michael L. Platt. "Neural Correlates of Reward and Attention in Macaque Area LIP." *Neuropsychologia* 44, no. 12 (2006): 2411–20.

Bennett, William J. *The Book of Virtues: A Treasury of Great Moral Stories*. New York: Simon & Schuster, 1993.

Berridge, Kent, and Morten Kringelbach. "Affective Neuroscience of Pleasure: Reward in Humans and Animals." *Psychopharmacology* 199, no. 3 (2008): 457–80.

Bester-Meredith, Janet K., and Catherine A. Marler. "Vasopressin and Aggression in Cross-Fostered California Mice (*Peromyscus californicus*) and White-Footed Mice (*Peromyscus leucopus*)." *Hormones and Behavior* 40, no. 1 (2001): 51–64.

Bishop, Jacqueline M, Colleen O'Ryan, and Jennifer U.M Jarvis. "Social Common Mole-Rats Enhance Outbreeding Via Extra-Pair Mating." *Biology Letters* 3, no. 2 (2007): 176–79.

Blackburn, Simon. *Ethics: A Very Short Introduction*. New York: Oxford University Press, 2003.

Blackburn, Simon. *How to Read Hume*. London: Granta, 2008.

Blackburn, Simon. "Response to Marc Hauser's Princeton Tanner Lecture." http://www.phil.cam.ac.uk/~swb24/PAPERS/Hauser.pdf, 2008.

Blair, R.J.R. "Neuroimaging of Psychopathy and Antisocial Behavior: A Targeted Review." *Current Psychiatry Reports* 12, no. 1 (2010): 76–82.

Blakemore, S.-J., D. Bristow, G. Bird, C. Frith, and J. Ward. "Somatosensory Activations During the Observation of Touch and a Case of Vision-Touch Synaesthesia." *Brain* 128, no. 7 (2005): 1571–83.

Boas, Franz. *The Central Eskimo*. Lincoln, NE: University of Nebraska Press, 1888/1964.

Boesch, Christophe, Camille Bolé, Nadin Eckhardt, and Hedwige Boesch. "Altruism in Forest Chimpanzees: The Case of Adoption." *PLoS ONE* 5, no. 1 (2010): e8901.

Bogaerts, Steven, and David Leake. "A Framework for Rapid and Modular Case-Based Reasoning System Development." Technical Report TR 617, Computer Science Department, Indiana University, Bloomington, Ind., 2005.

Bowles, Samuel. "Did Warfare among Ancestral Hunter-Gatherers Affect the Evolution of Human Social Behaviors?" *Science* 324, no. 5932 (2009): 1293–98.

Bowles, Samuel. "Group Competition, Reproductive Leveling, and the Evolution of Human Altruism." *Science* 314, no. 5805 (2006): 1569–72.

Boyd, Robert, and Peter J. Richerson. "Solving the Puzzle of Human Cooperation." In *Evolution and Culture*, edited by Stephen C. Levinson, 105–32. Cambridge, MA: MIT Press, 2005.

Boyer, Pascal. *Religion Explained: The Evolutionary Origins of Religious Thought*. New York: Basic Books, 2001.

Braver, Todd S., and Susan R. Bongiolatti. "The Role of Frontopolar Cortex in Sub-goal Processing During Working Memory." *Neuroimage* 15, no. 3 (2002): 523–36.

Brizendine, Louann. *The Female Brain*. New York: Morgan Road Books, 2006.

Brizendine, Louann. *The Male Brain*. New York: Broadway Books, 2010.

Broad, K. D., J. P. Curley, and E. B. Keverne. "Mother-Infant Bonding and the Evolution of Mammalian Social Relationships." *Philosophical Transactions of the Royal Society B: Biological Sciences* 361, no. 1476 (2006): 2199–214.

Brown, D.G. "Mill's Moral Theory: Ongoing Revisionism." *Politics, Philosophy & Economics* 9, no. 1 (2010): 5–45.

Bryson, Bill. *At Home: A Short History of Private Life*. New York: Doubleday, 2010.

Bulbulia, J., R. Sosis, E. Harris, R. Genet, C. Genet, and K. Wyman, eds. *The Evolution of Religion: Studies, Theories, and Critiques*. Santa Margarita, CA: Collins Foundation Press, 2008.

Buller, David J. "Four Fallacies of Pop Evolutionary Psychology." *Scientific American* 300 (2009): 74–81.

Bullmore, Ed, and Olaf Sporns. "Complex Brain Networks: Graph Theoretical Analysis of Structural and Functional Systems." *Nature Reviews Neuroscience* 10, no. 3 (2009): 186–98.

Burch, Ernest S. *Alliance and Conflict: The World System of the Iñupiaq Eskimos.* Lincoln: University of Nebraska Press, 2005.

Burkart, Judith M., Ernst Fehr, Charles Efferson, and Carel P. van Schaik. "Other-Regarding Preferences in a Non-Human Primate: Common Marmosets Provision Food Altruistically." *Proceedings of the National Academy of Sciences* 104, no. 50 (2007): 19762–66.

Buzsáki, G. *Rhythms of the Brain.* Oxford: Oxford University Press, 2006.

Caldwell, Christine A., and Ailsa E. Millen. "Social Learning Mechanisms and Cumulative Cultural Evolution." *Psychological Science* 20, no. 12 (2009): 1478–83.

Carroll, Robert P., and Stephen Prickett, eds. *The Bible: Authorized King James Version.* New York: Oxford University Press, 2008.

Carter, C. Sue, Angela J. Grippo, Hossein Pournajafi-Nazarloo, Michael G. Ruscio, and Stephen W. Porges. "Oxytocin, Vasopressin and Sociality." In *Progress in Brain Research 170: Advances in Vasopressin and Oxytocin: From Genes to Behaviour to Disease,* edited by Inga D. Neumann and Rainer Landgraf, 331–36. New York: Elsevier, 2008.

Carter, C. Sue., J. Harris, and Stephen W. Porges. Neural and Evolutionary Perspectives on Empathy. In *The Social Neuroscience of Empathy,* edited by J. Decety and W. Ickes, 169–82, Cambridge, MA: MIT Press, 2009.

Carter, C. Sue, H. Pournajafi-Nazarloo, K. M. Kramer, T. E. Ziegler, R. White-Traut, D. Bello, and D. Schwertz. "Oxytocin: behavioral associations and potential as a salivary biomarker." *Annals of the New York Academy of Sciences* 1098 (2007): 312–22.

Casebeer, William D. *Natural Ethical Facts: Evolution, Connectionism, and Moral Cognition.* Cambridge, MA: MIT Press, 2003.

Champagne, Frances A., and Michael J. Meaney. "Like Mother, Like Daughter: Evidence for Non-Genomic Transmission of Parental Behavior and Stress Responsivity." *Progress in Brain Research* 133 (2001): 287–302.

Champagne, Frances A., and Michael J. Meaney. "Transgenerational Effects of Social Environment on Variations in Maternal Care and Behavioral Response to Novelty." *Behavioral Neuroscience* 121, no. 6 (2007): 1353–63.

Chartrand, T. L., and J. A. Bargh. "The Chameleon Effect: The Perception-Behavior Link and Social Interaction." *Journal of Personality and Social Psychology* 76, no. 6 (1999): 893–910.

Cheney, Dorothy L., and Robert M. Seyfarth. *Baboon Metaphysics: The Evolution of a Social Mind.* Chicago: University of Chicago Press, 2007.

Cheng, Clara Michelle, and Tanya L. Chartrand. "Self-Monitoring without Awareness: Using Mimicry as a Nonconscious Affiliation Strategy." *Journal of Personality and Social Psychology* 85, no. 6 (2003): 1170–79.

Cheng, Yawei, Chenyi Chen, Ching-Po Lin, Kun-Hsien Chou, and Jean Decety. "Love Hurts: An fMRI Study." *Neuroimage* 51, no. 2 (2010): 923–29.

Cheng, Yawei, Ching-Po Lin, Ho-Ling Liu, Yuan-Yu Hsu, Kun-Eng Lim, Daisy Hung, and Jean Decety. "Expertise Modulates the Perception of Pain in Others." *Current Biology* 17, no. 19 (2007): 1708–13.

Choi, Jung-Kyoo, and Samuel Bowles. "The Coevolution of Parochial Altruism and War." *Science* 318, no. 5850 (2007): 636–40.

Christiansen, Morten H., and Nick Chater. "Language as Shaped by the Brain." *Behavioral and Brain Sciences* 31, no. 5 (2008): 489–509.

Churchland, Anne K., Roozbeh Kiani, and Michael N. Shadlen. "Decision-Making with Multiple Alternatives." *Nature Neuroscience* 11, no. 6 (2008): 693–702.

Churchland, Patricia S. "Human Dignity from a Neurophilosophical Perspective." In *Human Dignity and Bioethics: Essays Commissioned by the President's Council on Bioethics*, 99–121, Washington, DC: President's Council on Bioethics, 2008.

Churchland, Patricia S. "Inference to the Best Decision." In *The Oxford Handbook of Philosophy and Neuroscience*, edited by John Bickle, 419–30. New York: Oxford University Press, 2009.

Churchland, Paul M. "Rules, Know-How, and the Future of Moral Cognition." In *Moral Epistemology Naturalized*, edited by Richmond Campbell and Bruce Hunter, 291–306. Calgary: University of Calgary Press, 2000.

Churchland, Paul M. "Toward a Cognitive Neurobiology of the Moral Virtues." *Topoi* 17 (1998): 1–14.

Clayton, Nicola S., Joanna M. Dally, and Nathan J. Emery. "Social Cognition by Food-Caching Corvids: The Western Scrub-Jay as a Natural Psychologist." *Philosophical Transactions of the Royal Society B: Biological Sciences* 362, no. 1480 (2007): 507–22.

Clutton-Brock, Tim. "Cooperation between Non-Kin in Animal Societies." *Nature* 462, no. 7269 (2009): 51–57.

Cochran, Gregory, and Henry Harpending. *The 10,000 Year Explosion: How Civilization Accelerated Human Evolution*. New York: Basic Books, 2009.

Cohas, Aurélie, and Dominique Allainé. "Social Structure Influences Extra-Pair Paternity in Socially Monogamous Mammals." *Biology Letters* 5, no. 3 (2009): 313–16.

Collins, Francis S. *The Language of God: A Scientist Presents Evidence for Belief*. New York: Free Press, 2006.

Cordoni, G., and E. Palagi. "Reconciliation in Wolves (*Canis lupus*): New Evidence for a Comparative Perspective." *Ethology* 114, no. 3 (2008): 298–308.

Cosmides, Leda, John Tooby, and Jerome H. Barkow. "Introduction: Evolutionary Psychology and Conceptual Integration." In *The Adapted Mind: Evolutionary Psychology and the Generation of Culture*, ed. Jerome H. Barkow, Leda Cosmides, and John Tooby, 3–15. New York: Oxford University Press, 1992.

Craig, A. D. "How Do You Feel? Interoception: The Sense of the Physiological Condition of the Body." *Nature Reviews Neuroscience* 3, no. 8 (2002): 655–66.

Craig, A. D. "How Do You Feel—Now? The Anterior Insula and Human Awareness." *Nature Reviews Neuroscience* 10, no. 1 (2009): 59–70.

Craig, A. D. "Interoception and Emotion: A Neuroanatomical Perspective." In *Handbook of Emotions*, 3rd ed., edited by Michael Lewis, Jeannette M. Haviland-Jones, and Lisa F. Barrett, 272–88. New York: Guilford, 2008.

Craig, A. D. "A New View of Pain as a Homeostatic Emotion." *Trends in Neurosciences* 26, no. 6 (2003): 303–7.

Craig, A.D. "Pain Mechanisms: Labeled Lines versus Convergence in Central Processing." *Annual Review of Neuroscience* 26, no. 1 (2003): 1–30.

Craig A. D., K. Krout, and E. T. Zhang. "Cortical Projections of VMpo, a Specific Pain and Temperature Relay in Primate Thalamus." *Abstracts—Society for Neuroscience* 21 (1995): 1165.

Creel, Scott, and Nancy Marusha Creel. "Communal Hunting and Pack Size in African Wild Dogs, *Lycaon pictus*." *Animal Behaviour* 50, no. 5 (1995): 1325–39.

Crockett, M. J. "The Neurochemistry of Fairness." *Annals of the New York Academy of Sciences* 1167, no. 1 (2009): 76–86.

Crockett, M. J., L. Clark, G. Tabibnia, M. D. Lieberman, and T. W. Robbins. "Serotonin Modulates Behavioral Reactions to Unfairness." *Science* 320, no. 5884 (2008): 1739.

Damasio, Antonio R. *The Feeling of What Happens: Body and Emotion in the Making of Consciousness*. New York: Harcourt Brace, 1999.

Damasio, Antonio R. *Self Comes to Mind: Constructing the Conscious Brain*. New York: Knopf/Pantheon, 2010.

Dalrymple, William. *Nine Lives: In Search of the Sacred in Modern India*. London: Bloomsbury, 2009.

Danks, David. "Constraint-Based Human Causal Learning." In *Proceedings of the 6th International Conference on Cognitive Modeling (ICCM-2004)*, edited by M. Lovett, C. Schunn, C. Lebiere, and P. Munro, 342–43. Mahwah, NJ: Lawrence Erlbaum Associates, 2004.

Danks, David. "The Psychology of Causal Perception and Reasoning." In *The Oxford Handbook of Causation*, edited by H. Beebee, C. Hitchcock, and P. Menzies, 447–70. Oxford: Oxford University Press, 2009.

Dapretto, M., M. S. Davies, J. H. Pfeifer, A. A. Scott, M. Sigman, S. Y. Bookheimer, and M. Iacoboni. "Understanding Emotions in Others: Mirror Neuron Dysfunction in Children with Autism Spectrum Disorders." *Nature Neuroscience* 9, no. 1 (2006): 28–30.

Davila Ross, Marina, Susanne Menzler, and Elke Zimmermann. "Rapid Facial Mimicry in Orangutan Play." *Biology Letters* 4, no. 1 (2008): 27–30.

De Dreu, Carsten K. W., Lindred L. Greer, Michel J. J. Handgraaf, Shaul Shalvi, Gerben A. Van Kleef, Matthijs Baas, Femke S. Ten Velden, Eric Van Dijk, and Sander W. W. Feith. "The Neuropeptide Oxytocin Regulates Parochial Altruism in Intergroup Conflict among Humans." *Science* 328, no. 5984 (2010): 1408–11.

De Sousa, Ronald. *The Rationality of Emotion*. Cambridge, MA: MIT Press, 1987.

De Sousa, Ronald. *Why Think? Evolution and the Rational Mind*. Oxford: Oxford University Press, 2007.

de Waal, F.B.M., and K. E. Bonnie. "In Tune with Others: The Social Side of Primate Culture." In *The Question of Animal Culture*, edited by K. Laland and G. Galef, 19–39, Cambridge, MA: Harvard University Press, 2009.

Deaner, Robert O., Stephen V. Shepherd, and Michael L. Platt. "Familiarity Accentuates Gaze Cuing in Women but Not Men." *Biology Letters* 3, no. 1 (2007): 65–68.

Deary, Ian J., Lars Penke, and Wendy Johnson. "The Neuroscience of Human Intelligence Differences." *Nature Reviews Neuroscience* 11, no. 3 (2010): 201–11.

DeVries, A. Courtney, Tarra Guptaa, Serena Cardillo, Mary Cho, and C. Sue Carter. "Corticotropin-Releasing Factor Induces Social Preferences in Male Prairie Voles." *Psychoneuroendocrinology* 27, no. 6 (2002): 705–14.

Dierick, Herman A., and Ralph J. Greenspan. "Molecular Analysis of Flies Selected for Aggressive Behavior." *Nature Genetics* 38, no. 9 (2006): 1023–31.

Dierick, Herman A., and Ralph J. Greenspan. "Serotonin and Neuropeptide F Have Opposite Modulatory Effects on Fly Aggression." *Nat Genet* 39, no. 5 (2007): 678–82.

Domes, Gregor, M. Heinrichs, J. Glascher, C. Buchel, D. F. Braus, and S. C. Herpertz. "Oxytocin Attenuates Amygdala Responses to Emotional Faces Regardless of Valence." *Biological Psychiatry* 62, no. 10 (2007): 1187–90.

Domes, Gregor, Markus Heinrichs, Andre Michel, Christoph Berger, and Sabine C. Herpertz. "Oxytocin Improves 'Mind-Reading' in Humans." *Biological Psychiatry* 61, no. 6 (2007): 731–33.

Domes, Gregor, Alexander Lischke, Christoph Berger, Annette Grossmann, Karlheinz Hauenstein, Markus Heinrichs, and Sabine C. Herpertz. "Effects of Intranasal Oxytocin on Emotional Face Processing in Women." *Psychoneuroendocrinology* 35, no. 1 (2010): 83–93.

Dunbar, R.I.M. "Coevolution of Neocortical Size, Group Size and Language in Humans." *Behavioral and Brain Sciences* 16, no. 04 (1993): 681–94.

Dunbar, R.I.M. *Grooming, Gossip and the Evolution of Language*. London: Faber and Faber, 1996.

Dunham, A. E., and V.H.W. Rudolf. "Evolution of Sexual Size Monomorphism: The Influence of Passive Mate Guarding." *Journal of Evolutionary Biology* 22, no. 7 (2009): 1376–86.

Dupanloup, Isabelle, Luísa Pereira, Giorgio Bertorelle, Francesc Calafell, Maria João Prata, Antonio Amorim, and Guido Barbujani. "A Recent Shift from Polygyny to Monogamy in Humans Is Suggested by the Analysis of Worldwide Y-Chromosome Diversity." *Journal of Molecular Evolution* 57, no. 1 (2003): 85–97.

Eisenberger, Naomi I., and Matthew D. Lieberman. "Why Rejection Hurts: A Common Neural Alarm System for Physical and Social Pain." *Trends in Cognitive Sciences* 8, no. 7 (2004): 294–300.

Eisenberger, Naomi I., Matthew D. Lieberman, and Kipling D. Williams. "Does Rejection Hurt? An fMRI Study of Social Exclusion." *Science* 302, no. 5643 (2003): 290–92.

Elman, Jeffrey L., Elizabeth A. Bates, Mark H. Johnson, Annette Karmiloff-Smith, Domenico Parisi, and Kim Plunkett. *Rethinking Innateness: A Connectionist*

Perspective on Development, Neural Network Modeling and Connectionism. Cambridge, MA: MIT Press, 1996.

Emery, Nathan J., and Nicola S. Clayton. "Comparative Social Cognition." *Annual Review of Psychology* 60, no. 1 (2008): 87–113.

Erickson, Kirk I., Walter R. Boot, Chandramallika Basak, Mark B. Neider, Ruchika S. Prakash, Michelle W. Voss, Ann M. Graybiel, Daniel J. Simons, Monica Fabiani, Gabriele Gratton, and Arthur F. Kramer. "Striatal Volume Predicts Level of Video Game Skill Acquisition." *Cerebral Cortex* (2010): bhp293.

"Extending Trust." Editorial, *Nature Neuroscience* 13, no. 8 (2010): 905.

Evans, Nicholas, and Stephen C. Levinson. "The Myth of Language Universals: Language Diversity and Its Importance for Cognitive Science." *Behavioral and Brain Sciences* 32, no. 5 (2009): 429–48.

Fehr, Ernst, and Simon Gächter. "Altruistic Punishment in Humans." *Nature* 415, no. 6868 (2002): 137–40.

Fehr, Ernst, and Simon Gächter. "Cooperation and Punishment in Public Goods Experiments." *American Economic Review* 90 (2000): 980–94.

Fehr, Ernst, and Urs Fischbacher. "Third-Party Punishment and Social Norms." *Evolution and Human Behavior* 25, no. 2 (2004): 63–87.

Feldman, Ruth, Ilanit Gordon, and Orna Zagoory-Sharon, "The Cross-Generation Transmission of Oxytocin in Humans," *Hormones and Behavior* (in press).

Ferrari, Pier F., Elisabetta Visalberghi, Annika Paukner, Leonardo Fogassi, Angela Ruggiero, and Stephen J. Suomi. "Neonatal Imitation in Rhesus Macaques." *PLoS Biology* 4, no. 9 (2006): e302.

Fink, Sabine, Laurent Excoffier, and Gerald Heckel. "Mammalian Monogamy Is Not Controlled by a Single Gene." *Proceedings of the National Academy of Sciences* 103, no. 29 (2006): 10956–60.

Fink, Sheri. "The Deadly Choices at Memorial." *New York Times Magazine*, August 30, 2009.

Flanagan, Owen J. *The Really Hard Problem: Meaning in a Material World*. Cambridge, MA: MIT Press, 2007.

Flanagan, Owen J. *Varieties of Moral Personality: Ethics and Psychological Realism*. Cambridge, MA: Harvard University Press, 1991.

Flanagan, Owen, and Robert Anthony Williams. "What Does the Modularity of Morals Have to Do with Ethics? Four Moral Sprouts Plus or Minus a Few." *Topics in Cognitive Science* (in press).

Flint, Jonathan, Ralph J. Greenspan, and Kenneth S. Kendler. *How Genes Influence Behavior*. New York: Oxford University Press, 2010.

Fogassi, Leonardo, Pier Francesco Ferrari, Benno Gesierich, Stefano Rozzi, Fabian Chersi, and Giacomo Rizzolatti. "Parietal Lobe: From Action Organization to Intention Understanding." *Science* 308, no. 5722 (2005): 662–67.

Forbes, Chad E., and Jordan Grafman. "The Role of the Human Prefrontal Cortex in Social Cognition and Moral Judgment." *Annual Review of Neuroscience* 33, no. 1 (2010): 299–324.

Fortunato, L., and M. Archetti. "Evolution of Monogamous Marriage by Maximization of Inclusive Fitness." *Journal of Evolutionary Biology* 23, no. 1 (2010): 149–56.

Freedman, O., S. Ornstein, P. Boston, T. Amour, J. Seely, and B. M. Mount. "Spirituality, Religion and Health: A Critical Appraisal of the Larson Reports." *Annals (Royal College of Physicians and Surgeons of Canada)* 35 (2002): 89–93.

Friedman, Daniel. *Morals and Markets: An Evolutionary Account of the Modern World.* New York: Palgrave Macmillan, 2008.

Frith, Chris D. "Social Cognition." *Philosophical Transactions of the Royal Society B: Biological Sciences* 363, no. 1499 (2008): 2033–39.

Frith, Chris D., and Uta Frith. "The Neural Basis of Mentalizing." *Neuron* 50, no. 4 (2006): 531–34.

Fuster, Joaquin M. *The Prefrontal Cortex.* 4th ed. Boston: Academic Press, 2008.

Gallese, Vittorio. "Motor Abstraction: A Neuroscientific Account of How Action Goals and Intentions Are Mapped and Understood." *Psychological Research* 73, no. 4 (2009): 486–98.

Gallese, Vittorio, Luciano Fadiga, Leonardo Fogassi, and Giacomo Rizzolatti. "Action Recognition in the Premotor Cortex." *Brain* 119, no. 2 (1996): 593–609.

Gallese, Vittorio, and Alvin Goldman. "Mirror Neurons and the Simulation Theory of Mind-Reading." *Trends in Cognitive Sciences* 2, no. 12 (1998): 493–501.

Gazzola, Valeria, and Christian Keysers. "The Observation and Execution of Actions Share Motor and Somatosensory Voxels in All Tested Subjects: Single-Subject Analyses of Unsmoothed fMRI Data." *Cerebral Cortex* 19, no. 6 (2009): 1239–55.

Gentner, Dedre, Keith James Holyoak, and Boicho N. Kokinov. *The Analogical Mind: Perspectives from Cognitive Science.* Cambridge, MA: MIT Press, 2001.

Germonpré, Mietje, Mikhail V. Sablin, Rhiannon E. Stevens, Robert E. M. Hedges, Michael Hofreiter, Mathias Stiller, and Viviane R. Després. "Fossil Dogs and Wolves from Palaeolithic Sites in Belgium, the Ukraine and Russia: Osteometry, Ancient DNA and Stable Isotopes." *Journal of Archaeological Science* 36, no. 2 (2009): 473–90.

Gert, Bernard. "The Definition of Morality." In *The Stanford Encyclopedia of Philosophy* (Fall 2008 Edition), ed. Edward N. Zalta. http://plato.stanford.edu/entries/morality-definition/, 2008.

Gervais, Matthew, and David Sloan Wilson. "The Evolution and Functions of Laughter and Humor: A Synthetic Approach." *Quarterly Review of Biology* 80, no. 4 (2005): 395–430.

Gintis, Herbert. *The Bounds of Reason: Game Theory and the Unification of the Behavioral Sciences.* Princeton, NJ: Princeton University Press, 2009.

Gintis, Herbert, Samuel Bowles, Robert Boyd, and Ernst Fehr. *Moral Sentiments and Material Interests: The Foundations of Cooperation in Economic Life.* Cambridge, MA: MIT Press, 2004.

Goldberg, Elkhonon, and Dmitri Bougakov. "Goals, Executive Control, and Action." In *Cognition, Brain, and Consciousness: Introduction to Cognitive Neuroscience,* edited by Bernard J. Baars and Nicole M. Gage. London: Academic Press, 2007.

Goldman, Alvin I. *Simulating Minds: The Philosophy, Psychology, and Neuroscience of Mindreading*, Philosophy of Mind. New York: Oxford University Press, 2006.

Goldman, Alvin, and Frederique de Vignemont. "Is Social Cognition Embodied?" *Trends in Cognitive Sciences* 13, no. 4 (2009): 154–59.

Goodson, James L. "The Vertebrate Social Behavior Network: Evolutionary Themes and Variations." *Hormones and Behavior* 48, no. 1 (2005): 11–22.

Goodson, James L., Sara E. Schrock, James D. Klatt, David Kabelik, and Marcy A. Kingsbury. "Mesotocin and Nonapeptide Receptors Promote Estrildid Flocking Behavior." *Science* 325 (2009): 862–866.

Gopnik, Alison. "Mind Reading." Review of *Reading in the Brain — The Science and Evolution of a Human Invention*, by Stanislas Dehaene. *New York Times*, January 3, 2010.

Gottfried, Jay A., John O'Doherty, and Raymond J. Dolan. "Encoding Predictive Reward Value in Human Amygdala and Orbitofrontal Cortex." *Science* 301, no. 5636 (2003): 1104–7.

Gouin, Jean-Philippe, C. Sue Carter, Hossein Pournajafi-Nazarloo, Ronald Glaser, William B. Malarkey, Timothy J. Loving, Jeffrey Stowell, and Janice K. Kiecolt-Glaser. "Marital Behavior, Oxytocin, Vasopressin, and Wound Healing." *Psychoneuroendocrinology* (in press).

Grafton, Scott T., and Antonia F. de C. Hamilton. "Evidence for a Distributed Hierarchy of Action Representation in the Brain." *Human Movement Science* 26, no. 4 (2007): 590–616.

Graham, Franklin. *The Name*. Nashville, TN: Thomas Nelson Publishers, 2002.

Graham, Jesse, Jonathan Haidt, and Brian A. Nosek. "Liberals and Conservatives Rely on Different Sets of Moral Foundations." *Journal of Personality and Social Psychology* 96, no. 5 (2009): 1029–46.

Graybiel, Ann M. "The Basal Ganglia: Learning New Tricks and Loving It." *Current Opinion in Neurobiology* 15, no. 6 (2005): 638–44.

Graybiel, Ann M. "Habits, Rituals, and the Evaluative Brain." *Annual Review of Neuroscience* 31 (2008): 359–87.

Grayling, A. C. *What Is Good? The Search for the Best Way to Live*. London: Weidenfeld & Nicolson, 2003.

Greene, Joshua. "From Neural 'Is' to Moral 'Ought': What Are the Moral Implications of Neuroscientific Moral Psychology?" *Nature Reviews Neuroscience* 4, no. 10 (2003): 846–50.

Greenspan, R. J. "E Pluribus Unum, Ex Uno Plura: Quantitative and Single-Gene Perspectives on the Study of Behavior." *Annual Review of Neuroscience* 27 (2004): 79–105.

Greenspan, R. J. "The Flexible Genome." *Nature Reviews Genetics* 2, no. 5 (2001): 383–87.

Gross, Charles G. "Making Sense of Printed Symbols." *Science* 327, no. 5965 (2010): 524–25.

Gunter, T. D., M. G. Vaughn, and R. A. Philibert. "Behavioral Genetics in Antisocial Spectrum Disorders and Psychopathy: A Review of the Recent Literature." *Behavioral Sciences & the Law* 28, no. 2 (2010): 148–73.

Haidt, Jonathan. "The Emotional Dog and Its Rational Tail: A Social Intuitionist Approach to Moral Judgment." *Psychological Review* 108, no. 4 (2001): 814–34.

Haidt, Jonathan, and Jesse Graham. "Planet of the Durkheimians, Where Community, Authority, and Sacredness are Foundations of Morality." In *Social and Psychological Bases of Ideology and System Justification*, edited by John T. Jost, Aaron C. Kay, and Hulda Thorisdottir, 371–401. New York: Oxford University Press, 2009.

Haidt, Jonathan, and Craig Joseph. "Intuitive Ethics: How Innately Prepared Intuitions Generate Culturally Variable Virtues." *Daedalus*, 133, no. 4 (2004): 55–66.

Haidt, Jonathan, and Craig Joseph. "The Moral Mind: How Five Sets of Innate Intuitions Guide the Development of Many Culture-Specific Virtues, and Perhaps Even Modules." In *The Innate Mind*, vol. 3: *Foundations and the Future*, edited by Peter Carruthers, Stephen Laurence, and Stephen Stich, 367–92. New York: Oxford University Press, 2007.

Hanson, Stephen José, and Yaroslav O. Halchenko. "Brain Reading Using Full Brain Support Vector Machines for Object Recognition: There Is No 'Face' Identification Area." *Neural Computation* 20, no. 2 (2008): 486–503.

Hare, Brian. "What Is the Effect of Affect on Bonobo and Chimpanzee Problem Solving?" In *Neurobiology of "Umwelt": How Living Beings Perceive the World*, edited by Alain Berthoz and Yves Christen, 89–102. New York: Springer, 2009.

Hare, Brian, Alicia P. Melis, Vanessa Woods, Sara Hastings, and Richard Wrangham. "Tolerance Allows Bonobos to Outperform Chimpanzees on a Cooperative Task." *Current Biology* 17, no. 7 (2007): 619–23.

Hare, R. M. *Moral Thinking: Its Levels, Method, and Point.* Oxford: Clarendon Press, 1981.

Hare, Robert D. *Manual for the Hare Psychopathy Checklist-Revised, 2nd ed.* Toronto: Multi-Health Systems, 2003.

Hare, Robert D. *Without Conscience: The Disturbing World of the Psychopaths among Us.* New York: Pocket Books, 1993.

Hare, Robert D., and C. N. Neumann. "The PCL-R Assessment of Psychopathy: Development, Structural Properties, and New Directions." In *Handbook of Psychopathy*, edited by C. Patrick, 58–88. New York: Guilford, 2006.

Harris, Sam. *The Moral Landscape: How Science Can Determine Human Values.* New York: Free Press, 2010.

Harris, Sam. "Science Is in the Details." *New York Times*, July 26, 2009.

Hauser, Marc D. "Costs of Deception: Cheaters Are Punished in Rhesus Monkeys (*Macaca mulatta*)." *Proceedings of the National Academy of Sciences of the United States of America* 89, no. 24 (1992): 12137–39.

Hauser, Marc D. *Moral Minds: How Nature Designed Our Universal Sense of Right and Wrong.* New York: Ecco, 2006.

Haynes, John-Dylan, Katsuyuki Sakai, Geraint Rees, Sam Gilbert, Chris Frith, and Richard E. Passingham. "Reading Hidden Intentions in the Human Brain." *Current Biology* 17, no. 4 (2007): 323–28.

Heim, C., L. J. Young, D. J. Newport, T. Mletzko, A. H. Miller, and C. B. Nemeroff. "Lower Csf Oxytocin Concentrations in Women with a History of Childhood Abuse." *Molecular Psychiatry* 14, no. 10 (2008): 954–58.

Hein, Grit, and Tania Singer. "I Feel How You Feel but Not Always: The Empathic Brain and Its Modulation." *Current Opinion in Neurobiology* 18, no. 2 (2008): 153–58.

Heinrich, Bernd. *Mind of the Raven: Investigations and Adventures with Wolf-Birds.* New York: Cliff Street Books, 1999.

Heinrich, Bernd. *One Man's Owl.* Princeton, NJ: Princeton University Press, 1987.

Henrich, Joseph, Jean Ensminger, Richard McElreath, Abigail Barr, Clark Barrett, Alexander Bolyanatz, Juan Camilo Cardenas, Michael Gurven, Edwins Gwako, Natalie Henrich, Carolyn Lesorogol, Frank Marlowe, David Tracer, and John Ziker. "Markets, Religion, Community Size, and the Evolution of Fairness and Punishment." *Science* 327, no. 5972 (2010): 1480–84.

Henshilwood, Christopher S., Francesco D'Errico, Curtis W. Marean, Richard G. Milo, and Royden Yates. "An Early Bone Tool Industry from the Middle Stone Age at Blombos Cave, South Africa: Implications for the Origins of Modern Human Behaviour, Symbolism and Language." *Journal of Human Evolution* 41, no. 6 (2001): 631–78.

Henshilwood, Christopher S., Francesco d'Errico, Marian Vanhaeren, Karen van Niekerk, and Zenobia Jacobs. "Middle Stone Age Shell Beads from South Africa." *Science* 304 (2004): 404.

Heyes, Cecilia. "Where Do Mirror Neurons Come From?" *Neuroscience & Biobehavioral Reviews* 34, no. 4 (2010): 575–83.

Hickok, Gregory. "Eight Problems for the Mirror Neuron Theory of Action Understanding in Monkeys and Humans." *Journal of Cognitive Neuroscience* 21, no. 7 (2009): 1229–43.

Hickok, Gregory, Kayoko Okada, and John T. Serences. "Area SPT in the Human Planum Temporale Supports Sensory-Motor Integration for Speech Processing." *Journal of Neurophysiology* 101, no. 5 (2009): 2725–32.

Hoesch, W. "Uber Ziegen hutende Bärenpaviane (*Papio ursinus ruacana*)." *Zeitschrift für Tierpsychologie* (1961) 18: 297–301.

Hollander, Eric, Jennifer Bartz, William Chaplin, Ann Phillips, Jennifer Sumner, Latha Soorya, Evdokia Anagnostou, and Stacey Wasserman. "Oxytocin Increases Retention of Social Cognition in Autism." *Biological Psychiatry* 61 (2007): 498–503.

Holt-Lunstad, Julianne, Wendy A. Birmingham, and Kathleen C. Light. "Influence of a "Warm Touch" Support Enhancement Intervention among Married Couples on Ambulatory Blood Pressure, Oxytocin, Alpha Amylase, and Cortisol." *Psychosomatic Medicine* 70, no. 9 (2008): 976–85.

Horner, Victoria, and Frans B. M. de Waal. "Controlled Studies of Chimpanzee Cultural Transmission." *Progress in Brain Research* 178 (2009): 3–15.

Hrdy, Sarah Blaffer. *Mother Nature: A History of Mothers, Infants, and Natural Selection.* New York: Pantheon Books, 1999.

Hrdy, Sarah Blaffer. *Mothers and Others: The Evolutionary Origins of Mutual Understanding.* Cambridge, MA: Belknap Press of Harvard University Press, 2009.

Hughes, John R. "Update on Autism: A Review of 1300 Reports Published in 2008." *Epilepsy & Behavior* 16, no. 4 (2009): 569–89.

Hume, David. *A Treatise of Human Nature*, edited by David Fate Norton and Mary J. Norton. Oxford: Oxford University Press, 2000.

Hurka, Thomas "Moore's Moral Philosophy." In the *Stanford Encyclopedia of Philosophy*, ed. Edward M. Zalta. http://plato.stanford.edu/entries/moore-moral/, January 2005, with revisions in March 2010.

Hutchison, W. D., K. D. Davis, A. M. Lozano, R. R. Tasker, and J. O. Dostrovsky. "Pain-Related Neurons in the Human Cingulate Cortex." *Nature Neuroscience* 2, no. 5 (1999): 403–5.

Iacoboni, Marco. *Mirroring People: The New Science of How We Connect with Others*. New York: Farrar, Straus and Giroux, 2008.

Iacoboni, Marco. "Neurobiology of Imitation." *Current Opinion in Neurobiology* 19, no. 6 (2009): 661–65.

Iacoboni, Marco, Istvan Molnar-Szakacs, Vittorio Gallese, Giovanni Buccino, John C. Mazziotta, and Giacomo Rizzolatti. "Grasping the Intentions of Others with One's Own Mirror Neuron System." *PLoS Biology* 3, no. 3 (2005): e79.

Insel, Thomas R. "The Challenge of Translation in Social Neuroscience: A Review of Oxytocin, Vasopressin, and Affiliative Behavior." *Neuron* 65, no. 6 (2010): 768–79.

Jabbi, Mbemba, and Christian Keysers. "Inferior Frontal Gyrus Activity Triggers Anterior Insula Response to Emotional Facial Expressions." *Emotion* 8 (2008): 775–80.

Jacob, Pierre. "What Do Mirror Neurons Contribute to Human Social Cognition?" *Mind & Language* 23, no. 2 (2008): 190–223.

Jacob, Pierre, and Marc Jeannerod. "The Motor Theory of Social Cognition: A Critique." *Trends in Cognitive Sciences* 9, no. 1 (2005): 21–25.

Jahfari, Sara, Cathy M. Stinear, Mike Claffey, Frederick Verbruggen, and Adam R. Aron. "Responding with Restraint: What Are the Neurocognitive Mechanisms?" *Journal of Cognitive Neuroscience* 22, no. 7 (2010): 1479–92.

Jamieson, Dale. "When Utilitarians Should Be Virtue Theorists." *Utilitas* 19, no. 2 (2007): 160–83.

Johansson, Petter, Lars Hall, Sverker Sikstrom, and Andreas Olsson. "Failure to Detect Mismatches between Intention and Outcome in a Simple Decision Task." *Science* 310, no. 5745 (2005): 116–19.

Johnson, Dominic. "Darwinian Selection in Asymmetric Warfare: The Natural Advantage of Insurgents and Terrorists." *Journal of the Washington Academy of Sciences* 95 (2009): 89–112.

Johnson, Mark. *Moral Imagination: Implications of Cognitive Science for Ethics*. Chicago: University of Chicago Press, 1993.

Johnson, Robert. "Kant's Moral Philosophy." In *The Stanford Encyclopedia of Philosophy (Winter 2009 Edition)*, edited by Edward N. Zalta. http://plato.stanford.edu/archives/win2009/entries/kant-moral, 2008.

Jones, Susan S. "Imitation in Infancy." *Psychological Science* 18, no. 7 (2007): 593–99.

Jones, Susan S. "Infants Learn to Imitate by Being Imitated." In *Proceedings of the International Conference on Development and Learning (ICDL)*, edited by C. Yu, L. B. Smith, and O. Sporns. Bloomington: Indiana University, 2006.

Jones, Susan S. "The Role of Mirror Neurons in Imitation: A Commentary on Gallese." In *Perspectives on Imitation: From Neuroscience to Social Science*, vol. 1:

Mechanisms of Imitation and Imitation in Animals, edited by Susan Hurley and Nick Chater, 205–210. Cambridge, MA: MIT Press, 2005.

Kant, Immanuel. *Groundwork of the Metaphysics of Morals*, edited by Mary J. Gregor. New York: Cambridge University Press, 1998.

Kaplan, Jonathan Michael. "Historical Evidence and Human Adaptations." *Philosophy of Science* 69, no. s3 (2002): S294–S304.

Kavanagh, L., C. Suhler, P. Churchland, and P. Winkielman. "People who mimic unfriendly individuals suffer reputational costs" (submitted).

Kehagia, Angie A., Graham K. Murray, and Trevor W. Robbins. "Learning and Cognitive Flexibility: Frontostriatal Function and Monoaminergic Modulation." *Current Opinion in Neurobiology* 20, no. 2 (2010): 199–204.

Keverne, Eric B. "Central Mechanisms Underlying the Neural and Neuroendocrine Determinants of Maternal Behaviour." *Psychoneuroendocrinology* 13, no. 1–2 (1988): 127–41.

Keverne, Eric B. "Genomic Imprinting and the Evolution of Sex Differences in Mammalian Reproductive Strategies." *Advances in Genetics* 59 (2007): 217–43.

Keverne, Eric B. "Reproductive Behaviour." In *Reproduction in Mammals*, vol. 4: *Reproductive Fitness*, edited by C. R. Austin and R. V. Short, 133–75. Cambridge: Cambridge University Press, 1984.

Keverne, Eric B. "Understanding Well-Being in the Evolutionary Context of Brain Development." *Philosophical Transactions of the Royal Society of London B: Biological Sciences* 359, no. 1449 (2004): 1349–58.

Keverne, Eric B., and K. M. Kendrick. "Neurochemical Changes Accompanying Parturition and Their Significance for Maternal Behavior." In *Mammalian Parenting: Biochemical, Neurobiological and Behavioral Determinants*, edited by N. A. Krasnegor and R. S. Bridges, 281–304. New York: Oxford University Press, 1990.

Keysers, Christian, and Valeria Gazzola. "Towards a Unifying Neural Theory of Social Cognition." *Progress in Brain Research* 156 (2006): 379–401.

Keysers, Christian, Jon H. Kaas, and Valeria Gazzola. "Somatosensation in Social Perception." *Nature Reviews Neuroscience* 11, no. 6 (2010): 417–28.

Keysers, Christian, and David I. Perrett. "Demystifying Social Cognition: A Hebbian Perspective." *Trends in Cognitive Sciences* 8, no. 11 (2004): 501–7.

Kiehl, Kent A. "A Cognitive Neuroscience Perspective on Psychopathy: Evidence for Paralimbic System Dysfunction." *Psychiatry Research* 142 (2006): 107–28.

Kilham, Benjamin, and Ed Gray. *Among the Bears: Raising Orphan Cubs in the Wild.* New York: Henry Holt, 2002.

King-Casas, B., C. Sharp, L. Lomax-Bream, T. Lohrenz, P. Fonagy, and P. R. Montague. "The Rupture and Repair of Cooperation in Borderline Personality Disorder." *Science* 321, no. 5890 (2008): 806–10.

Kirsch, P., C. Esslinger, Q. Chen, D. Mier, S. Lis, S. Siddhanti, H. Gruppe, V. S. Mattay, B. Gallhofer, and A. Meyer-Lindenberg. "Oxytocin Modulates Neural Circuitry for Social Cognition and Fear in Humans." *The Journal of Neuroscience* 25, no. 49 (2005): 11489–93.

Kitcher, Philip. "Biology and Ethics." In *The Oxford Handbook of Ethics*, edited by D. Copp, 163–85. Oxford: Oxford University Press, 2006.

Kleiman, Devra G. "Monogamy in Mammals." *Quarterly Review of Biology* 52, no. 1 (1977): 39–69.

Kline, Michelle A., and Robert Boyd. "Population Size Predicts Technological Complexity in Oceania." *Proceedings of the Royal Society B: Biological Sciences* 277, no. 1693 (2010): 2559–64.

Korsgaard, Christine M. *The Sources of Normativity*. New York: Cambridge University Press, 1996.

Kosfeld, M., M. Heinrichs, P. J. Zak, U. Fischbacher, and E. Fehr. "Oxytocin Increases Trust in Humans." *Nature* 435, no. 7042 (2005): 673–76.

Krubitzer, Leah. "The Magnificent Compromise: Cortical Field Evolution in Mammals." *Neuron* 56 (2007): 201–9.

La Cerra, Peggy, and Roger Bingham. *The Origin of Minds: Evolution, Uniqueness, and the New Science of the Self*. New York: Harmony Books, 2002.

Lakin, Jessica L., and T. L. Chartrand. "Using Nonconscious Behavioral Mimicry to Create Affiliation and Rapport." *Psychological Science* 14, no. 4 (2003): 334–39.

Lakin, Jessica L., Valerie E. Jefferis, Clara Michelle Cheng, and Tanya L. Chartrand. "The Chameleon Effect as Social Glue: Evidence for the Evolutionary Significance of Nonconscious Mimicry." *Journal of Nonverbal Behavior* 27, no. 3 (2003): 145–62.

Lakoff, George, and Mark Johnson. *Philosophy in the Flesh: The Embodied Mind and Its Challenge to Western Thought*. New York: Basic Books, 1999.

Larson, David B., James P. Swyers, and Michael E. McCullough. *Scientific Research on Spirituality and Health: A Report Based on the Scientific Progress in Spirituality Conferences*. Rockville, MD: National Institute for Healthcare Research, 1998.

Leake, David B. *Case-Based Reasoning: Experiences, Lessons and Future Directions*. Cambridge, MA: MIT Press, 1996.

Lesch, Klaus-Peter, Dietmar Bengel, Armin Heils, Sue Z. Sabol, Benjamin D. Greenberg, Susanne Petri, Jonathan Benjamin, Clemens R. Muller, Dean H. Hamer, and Dennis L. Murphy. "Association of Anxiety-Related Traits with a Polymorphism in the Serotonin Transporter Gene Regulatory Region." *Science* 274, no. 5292 (1996): 1527–31.

Light, Kathleen C., Karen M. Grewen, Janet A. Amico, Maria Boccia, Kimberly A. Brownley, and Josephine M. Johns. "Deficits in Plasma Oxytocin Responses and Increased Negative Affect, Stress, and Blood Pressure in Mothers with Cocaine Exposure During Pregnancy." *Addictive Behaviors* 29, no. 8 (2004): 1541–64.

Lim, Miranda M., Anne Z. Murphy, and Larry J. Young. "Ventral Striatopallidal Oxytocin and Vasopressin V1a Receptors in the Monogamous Prairie Vole (*Microtus ochrogaster*)." *Journal of Comparative Neurology* 468, no. 4 (2004): 555–70.

Llinás, Rodolfo R. *I of the Vortex: From Neurons to Self*. Cambridge, MA: MIT Press, 2001.

Lucki, Irwin. "The Spectrum of Behaviors Influenced by Serotonin." *Biological Psychiatry* 44, no. 3 (1998): 151–62.

Lyons, Derek E., Andrew G. Young, and Frank C. Keil. "The Hidden Structure of Overimitation." *Proceedings of the National Academy of Sciences* 104, no. 50 (2007): 19751–56.

MacIntyre, Alasdair C. *After Virtue: A Study in Moral Theory.* 3rd ed. Notre Dame, IN: University of Notre Dame Press, 2007.

MacLean, Paul D. *The Triune Brain in Evolution: Role in Paleocerebral Functions.* New York: Plenum Press, 1990.

Maestripieri, Dario, Christy L. Hoffman, George M. Anderson, C. Sue Carter, and James D. Higley. "Mother-Infant Interactions in Free-Ranging Rhesus Macaques: Relationships between Physiological and Behavioral Variables." *Physiology & Behavior* 96, no. 4–5 (2009): 613–19.

Marean, Curtis W. "When the Sea Saved Humanity." *Scientific American* 303 (2010): 55–61.

McBrearty, Sally, and Alison S. Brooks. "The Revolution That Wasn't: A New Interpretation of the Origin of Modern Human Behavior." *Journal of Human Evolution* 39, no. 5 (2000): 453–563.

McGrew, William C. "Chimpanzee Technology." *Science* 328, no. 5978 (2010): 579–80.

McIntosh, Daniel N., Aimee Reichmann-Decker, Piotr Winkielman, and Julia L. Wilbarger. "When the Social Mirror Breaks: Deficits in Automatic, but Not Voluntary, Mimicry of Emotional Facial Expressions in Autism." *Developmental Science* 9, no. 3 (2006): 295–302.

Meaney, Michael J. "Maternal Care, Gene Expression, and the Transmission of Individual Differences in Stress Reactivity across Generations." *Annual Review of Neuroscience* 24, no. 1 (2003): 1161–92.

Melis, Alicia P., Brian Hare, and Michael Tomasello. "Engineering Cooperation in Chimpanzees: Tolerance Constraints on Cooperation." *Animal Behaviour* 72, no. 2 (2006): 275–86.

Mello, Claudio V., Tarciso A. F. Velho, and Raphael Pinaud. "Song-Induced Gene Expression: A Window on Song Auditory Processing and Perception." *Annals of the New York Academy of Sciences* 1016 (2004): 263–81.

Meltzoff, A. N. "Roots of Social Cognition: The Like-Me Framework." In *Minnesota Symposia on Child Psychology: Meeting the Challenge of Translational Research in Child Psychology,* edited by D. Cicchetti and M. R. Gunnar, 29–58. Hoboken, NJ: Wiley, 2009.

Meng, Qingjin, Jinyuan Liu, David J. Varricchio, Timothy Huang, and Chunling Gao. "Palaeontology: Parental Care in an Ornithischian Dinosaur." *Nature* 431, no. 7005 (2004): 145–46.

Mercier, Hugo, and Dan Sperber. "Why Do Humans Reason? Arguments for an Argumentative Theory." *Behavioral and Brain Sciences* (in press).

Mesoudi, Alex. "How Cultural Evolutionary Theory Can Inform Social Psychology and Vice Versa. " *Psychological Review,* no. 116 (2009): 929-952.

Meyer, Kaspar, and Antonio Damasio. "Convergence and Divergence in a Neural Architecture for Recognition and Memory." *Trends in Neurosciences* 32, no. 7 (2009): 376–82.

Milinski, M., D. Semmann, and H. J. Krambeck. "Reputation Helps Solve the 'Tragedy of the Commons.'" *Nature* 415, no. 6870 (2002): 424–26.

Mill, John Stuart. *Utilitarianism*. In *On Liberty and Other Essays*, edited by John Gray, 129–201, New York: Oxford University Press, 1998.

Molenberghs, Pascal, Ross Cunnington, and Jason B. Mattingley. "Is the Mirror Neuron System Involved in Imitation? A Short Review and Meta-Analysis." *Neuroscience & Biobehavioral Reviews* 33, no. 7 (2009): 975–80.

Moore, G. E. *Principia Ethica*. Cambridge: Cambridge University Press, 1903.

Morrison, India, and Paul E. Downing. "Organization of Felt and Seen Pain Responses in Anterior Cingulate Cortex." *Neuroimage* 37, no. 2 (2007): 642–51.

Murdock, George P., and Suzanne F. Wilson. "Settlement Patterns and Community Organization: Cross-Cultural Codes 3." *Ethnology* 11 (1972): 254–95.

Murphy, Dennis L., Meredith A. Fox, Kiara R. Timpano, Pablo R. Moya, Renee Ren-Patterson, Anne M. Andrews, Andrew Holmes, Klaus-Peter Lesch, and Jens R. Wendland. "How the Serotonin Story Is Being Rewritten by New Gene-Based Discoveries Principally Related to Slc6a4, the Serotonin Transporter Gene, Which Functions to Influence All Cellular Serotonin Systems." *Neuropharmacology* 55, no. 6 (2008): 932–60.

Murphy, Michael R., Jonathan R. Seckl, Steven Burton, Stuart A. Checkley, and Stafford L. Lightman. "Changes in Oxytocin and Vasopressin Secretion During Sexual Activity in Men." *The Journal of Clinical Endocrinology & Metabolism* 65, no. 4 (1987): 738–41.

Murray, Michael J., and Lyn Moore. "Costly Signaling and the Origin of Religion." *Journal of Cognition and Culture* 9 (2009): 225–45.

Myowa-Yamakoshi, Masako, Masaki Tomonaga, Masayuki Tanaka, and Tetsuro Matsuzawa. "Imitation in Neonatal Chimpanzees (*Pan troglodytes*)." *Developmental Science* 7, no. 4 (2004): 437–42.

Nagel, Thomas. "What Peter Singer Wants of You." *New York Review of Books*, March 25, 2010.

Neiman, Susan. *Moral Clarity: A Guide for Grown-up Idealists*. Orlando, FL: Harcourt, 2008.

Nesse, Randolph M. "Runaway Social Selection for Displays of Partner Value and Altruism." *Biological Theory* 2, no. 2 (2007): 143–55.

Nisbett, Richard E. *The Geography of Thought : How Asians and Westerners Think Differently—and Why*. New York: Free Press, 2003.

Nisbett, Richard E., and Dov Cohen. *Culture of Honor: The Psychology of Violence in the South*, New Directions in Social Psychology. Boulder, CO: Westview Press, 1996.

Nisbett, Richard E., and Timothy D. Wilson. "Telling More Than We Can Know: Verbal Reports on Mental Processes." *Psychological Review* 8 (1977): 231–59.

North, Douglass C., John Joseph Wallis, and Barry R. Weingast, *Violence and Social Orders: A Conceptual Framework for Interpreting Recorded Human History*, Cambridge: Cambridge University Press, 2009.

Oberman, Lindsay M., Edward M. Hubbard, Joseph P. McCleery, Eric L. Altschuler, Vilayanur S. Ramachandran, and Jaime A. Pineda. "EEG Evidence for Mirror

Neuron Dysfunction in Autism Spectrum Disorders." *Cognitive Brain Research* 24, no. 2 (2005): 190–98.

Oberman, Lindsay M., Jaime A. Pineda, and Vilayanur S. Ramachandran. "The Human Mirror Neuron System: A Link between Action Observation and Social Skills." *Social Cognitive and Affective Neuroscience* 2, no. 1 (2007): 62–66.

Oberman, Lindsay M., Piotr Winkielman, and Vilayanur S. Ramachandran. "Face to Face: Blocking Facial Mimicry Can Selectively Impair Recognition of Emotional Expressions." *Social Neuroscience* 2, no. 3–4 (2007): 167–78.

Olff, Miranda, Willie Langeland, Anke Witteveen, and Damiaan Denys. "A Psychobiological Rationale for Oxytocin in Treatment of Posttraumatic Stress Disorder." *CNS Spectrums* 15, no. 8 (2010): 436–44.

Ozonoff, Sally, Bruce F. Pennington, and Sally J. Rogers. "Executive Function Deficits in High-Functioning Autistic Individuals: Relationship to Theory of Mind." *Journal of Child Psychology and Psychiatry* 32, no. 7 (1991): 1081–105.

Oztop, Erhan, Mitsuo Kawato, and Michael Arbib. "Mirror Neurons and Imitation: A Computationally Guided Review." *Neural Networks* 19, no. 3 (2006): 254–71.

Pacheco, Jorge M., Francisco C. Santos, and Fabio A. C. C. Chalub. "Stern-Judging: A Simple, Successful Norm Which Promotes Cooperation under Indirect Reciprocity." *PLoS Computational Biology* 2, no. 12 (2006): e178.

Panksepp, Jaak. *Affective Neuroscience: The Foundations of Human and Animal Emotions*, Series in Affective Science. New York: Oxford University Press, 1998.

Panksepp, Jaak. "At the Interface of the Affective, Behavioral, and Cognitive Neurosciences: Decoding the Emotional Feelings of the Brain." *Brain and Cognition* 52, no. 1 (2003): 4–14.

Panksepp, Jaak. "Feeling the Pain of Social Loss." *Science* 302, no. 5643 (2003): 237–39.

Pargament, Kenneth I., Harold G. Koenig, Nalini Tarakeshwar, and June Hahn. "Religious Struggle as a Predictor of Mortality among Medically Ill Elderly Patients: A 2-Year Longitudinal Study." *Archives of Internal Medicine* 161, no. 15 (2001): 1881–85.

Parvizi, Josef. "Corticocentric Myopia: Old Bias in New Cognitive Sciences." *Trends in Cognitive Sciences* 13, no. 8 (2009): 354–59.

Pellegrino, G., L. Fadiga, L. Fogassi, V. Gallese, and G. Rizzolatti. "Understanding Motor Events: A Neurophysiological Study." *Experimental Brain Research* 91, no. 1 (1992): 176–80.

Pennisi, Elizabeth. "Conquering by Copying." *Science* 328, no. 5975 (2010): 165–67.

Pennisi, Elizabeth. "On the Origin of Cooperation." *Science* 325, no. 5945 (2009): 1196–99.

Perry, Susan, and Joseph H. Manson. "Traditions in Monkeys." *Evolutionary Anthropology: Issues, News, and Reviews* 12, no. 2 (2003): 71–81.

Perry, Susan, Joseph H. Manson, Gayle Dower, and Eva Wikberg. "White-faced Capuchins Cooperate to Rescue a Groupmate from a *Boa constrictor*." *Folia Primatologica* 74 (2003): 109–11.

Petit, Odile, Christine Desportes, and Bernard Thierry. "Differential Probability of 'Coproduction' in Two Species of Macaque (*Macaca tonkeana, M. mulatta*)." *Ethology* 90, no. 2 (1992): 107–20.

Pfaff, Donald W. *The Neuroscience of Fair Play: Why We (Usually) Follow the Golden Rule.* New York: Dana Press, 2007.

Phelps, Elizabeth A., Mauricio R. Delgado, Katherine I. Nearing, and Joseph E. LeDoux. "Extinction Learning in Humans: Role of the Amygdala and vmPFC." *Neuron* 43, no. 6 (2004): 897–905.

Poldrack, Russell A., Yaroslav O. Halchenko, and Stephen José Hanson. "Decoding the Large-Scale Structure of Brain Function by Classifying Mental States across Individuals." *Psychological Science* 20, no. 11 (2009): 1364–72.

Popper, Karl R. *Conjectures and Refutations: The Growth of Scientific Knowledge.* London: Routledge, 1963.

Porges, Stephen W. "The Polyvagal Perspective." *Biological Psychology* 74, no. 2 (2007): 116–43.

Porges, Stephen W., and C. Sue Carter. "Neurobiology and Evolution: Mechanisms, Mediators, and Adaptive Consequences of Caregiving." In *Self Interest and Beyond: Toward a New Understanding of Human Caregiving*, edited by S. L. Brown, R. M. Brown, and L. A. Penner. Oxford: Oxford University Press, in press.

Powell, Adam, Stephen Shennan, and Mark G. Thomas. "Late Pleistocene Demography and the Appearance of Modern Human Behavior." *Science* 324, no. 5932 (2009): 1298–301.

Preston, Stephanie D., and Frans B. M. de Waal. "Empathy: Its Ultimate and Proximate Bases." *Behavioral and Brain Sciences* 25, no. 1 (2001): 1–20.

Preuss, Todd M. "The Cognitive Neuroscience of Human Uniqueness." In *The Cognitive Neurosciences*, edited by M. S. Gazzaniga, 49–64. Cambridge, MA: MIT Press, 2009.

Preuss, Todd M. "Evolutionary Specializations of Primate Brain Systems." In *Primate Origins and Adaptations*, edited by M. J. Ravoso and M. Dagosto, 625–75. New York: Kluwer Academic/Plenum Press: 2007.

Preuss, Todd M. "Primate Brain Evolution in Phylogenetic Context." In *Evolution of Nervous Systems: A Comprehensive Reference*, vol. 4, edited by Jon H. Kaas and Todd M. Preuss, 1–34. Amsterdam: Academic Press, 2007.

Quartz, Steven, and Terrence J. Sejnowski. *Liars, Lovers, and Heroes: What the New Brain Science Reveals about How We Become Who We Are.* New York: William Morrow, 2002.

Raine, A., S. S. Ishikawa, E. Arce, T. Lencz, K. H. Knuth, S. Bihrle, L. LaCasse, and P. Colletti. "Hippocampal Structural Asymmetry in Unsuccessful Psychopaths." *Biological Psychiatry* 552 (2004): 185–91.

Rawls, John. *A Theory of Justice.* Oxford: Clarendon Press, 1972.

Raymaekers, Ruth, Jan Roelf Wiersema, and Herbert Roeyers. "EEG Study of the Mirror Neuron System in Children with High Functioning Autism." *Brain Research* 1304 (2009): 113–21.

Remnick, David. *Lenin's Tomb: The Last Days of the Soviet Empire.* New York: Random House, 1993.

Richardson, Robert C. *Evolutionary Psychology as Maladapted Psychology.* Cambridge, MA: MIT Press, 2007.

Richerson, Peter J., and Robert Boyd. *Not by Genes Alone: How Culture Transformed Human Evolution*. Chicago: University of Chicago Press, 2005.

Richerson, Peter J., Robert Boyd, and Joseph Henrich. "Gene-Culture Coevolution in the Age of Genomics." *Proceedings of the National Academy of Sciences* 107, Supplement 2 (2010): 8985–92.

Ridley, Matt. *The Rational Optimist*. New York: Harper Collins, 2010.

Rizzolatti, Giacomo, and Laila Craighero. "The Mirror-Neuron System." *Annual Review of Neuroscience* 27, no. 1 (2004): 169–92.

Rizzolatti, Giacomo, and Maddalena Fabbri-Destro. "Mirror Neurons: From Discovery to Autism." *Experimental Brain Research* 200, no. 3 (2010): 223–37.

Robbins, T. W., and A.F.T. Arnsten. "The Neuropsychopharmacology of Fronto-Executive Function: Monoaminergic Modulation." *Annual Review of Neuroscience* 32, no. 1 (2009): 267–87.

Roberts, A. C., Trevor W. Robbins, and Lawrence Weiskrantz. *The Prefrontal Cortex: Executive and Cognitive Functions*. New York: Oxford University Press, 1998.

Rockenbach, Bettina, and Manfred Milinski. "The Efficient Interaction of Indirect Reciprocity and Costly Punishment." *Nature* 444, no. 7120 (2006): 718–23.

Rodrigues, Sarina M., Laura R. Saslow, Natalia Garcia, Oliver P. John, and Dacher Keltner. "Oxytocin Receptor Genetic Variation Relates to Empathy and Stress Reactivity in Humans." *Proceedings of the National Academy of Sciences* 106, no. 50 (2009): 21437–41.

Roser, Matthew, and Michael S. Gazzaniga. "Automatic Brains—Interpretive Minds." *Current Directions in Psychological Science* 13, no. 2 (2004): 56–59.

Roskies, Adina. "Neuroimaging and Inferential Distance." *Neuroethics* 1, no. 1 (2008): 19–30.

Rue, Loyal D. *Religion Is Not About God: How Spiritual Traditions Nurture Our Biological Nature and What to Expect When They Fail*. New Brunswick, NJ: Rutgers University Press, 2005.

Sapolsky, Robert M. *A Primate's Memoir*. New York: Scribner, 2001.

Saxe, Rebecca. "The Neural Evidence for Simulation Is Weaker Than I Think You Think It Is." *Philosophical Studies* 144, no. 3 (2009): 447–56.

Scanlon, Thomas. *The Difficulty of Tolerance: Essays in Political Philosophy*. New York: Cambridge University Press, 2003.

Schaler, Jeffrey A., ed. *Peter Singer under Fire: The Moral Iconoclast Faces His Critics*. Chicago: Open Court, 2009.

Seed, Amanda M., Nicola S. Clayton, and Nathan J. Emery. "Postconflict Third-Party Affiliation in Rooks, *Corvus frugilegus*." *Current Biology* 17, no. 2 (2007): 152–58.

Seitz, Aaron R., Athanassios Protopapas, Yoshiaki Tsushima, Eleni L. Vlahou, Simone Gori, Stephen Grossberg, and Takeo Watanabe. "Unattended Exposure to Components of Speech Sounds Yields Same Benefits as Explicit Auditory Training." *Cognition* 115, no. 3 (2010): 435–43.

Sha, Ky. "A Mechanistic View of Genomic Imprinting." *Annual Review of Genomics and Human Genetics* 9, no. 1 (2008): 197–216.

Shumyatsky, Gleb P., Evgeny Tsvetkov, Gaël Malleret, Svetlana Vronskaya, Michael Hatton, Lori Hampton, James F. Battey, Catherine Dulac, Eric R. Kandel, and Vadim Y. Bolshakov. "Identification of a Signaling Network in Lateral Nucleus of Amygdala Important for Inhibiting Memory Specifically Related to Learned Fear." *Cell* 111, no. 6 (2002): 905–18.

Siever, Larry J. "Neurobiology of Aggression and Violence." *American Journal of Psychiatry* 165, no. 4 (2008): 429–42.

Singer, Peter. *Animal Liberation: A New Ethics for Our Treatment of Animals.* New York: Random House, 1975.

Singer, Peter. *Practical Ethics.* New York: Cambridge University Press, 1979.

Edward Slingerland, "Toward an Empirically Responsible Ethics: Cognitive Science, Virtue Ethics and Effortless Attention in Early Chinese Thought, " in *Effortless Attention: A New Perspective in the Cognitive Science of Attention and Action,* ed. Brian Bruya, 247–86. Cambridge, MA: MIT Press, 2010.

Solomon, Robert C. *Introducing Philosophy: A Text with Integrated Readings.* 9th ed. New York: Oxford University Press, 2008.

Sommer, Marc A., and Robert H. Wurtz. "Brain Circuits for the Internal Monitoring of Movements." *Annual Review of Neuroscience* 31, no. 1 (2008): 317–38.

Sosis, R., and C. Alcorta. "Signaling, Solidarity, and the Sacred: The Evolution of Religious Behavior." *Evolutionary Anthropology: Issues, News, and Reviews* 12, no. 6 (2003): 264–74.

Souter, David. "Commencement Address to Harvard University." http://news.harvard .edu/gazette/story/2010/05/text-of-justice-david-souters-speech/, Spring 2010.

Spunt, Robert P., Ajay B. Satpute, and Matthew D. Lieberman. "Identifying the What, Why, and How of an Observed Action: An fMRI Study of Mentalizing and Mechanizing During Action Observation." *Journal of Cognitive Neuroscience* (2010): 1–12.

Stout, Martha. *The Sociopath Next Door: The Ruthless Versus the Rest of Us.* New York: Broadway Books, 2005.

Striedter, Georg F. "Précis of *Principles of Brain Evolution.*" *Behavioral and Brain Sciences* 29, no. 1 (2006): 1–12.

Suhler, Christopher L., and Patricia S. Churchland. "Can Innate, Modular 'Foundations' Explain Morality? Challenges for Haidt's Moral Foundations Theory." *Journal of Cognitive Neuroscience* (forthcoming).

Suhler, Christopher L., and Patricia S. Churchland. "Control: Conscious and Otherwise." *Trends in Cognitive Sciences* 13, no. 8 (2009): 341–47.

Suhler, Christopher L., and Patricia S. Churchland. "The Neurobiological Basis of Morality." In *The Oxford Handbook of Neuroethics,* edited by Judy Illes and Barbara J. Sahakian, Oxford: Oxford University Press.

Talmi, Deborah, Peter Dayan, Stefan J. Kiebel, Chris D. Frith, and Raymond J. Dolan. "How Humans Integrate the Prospects of Pain and Reward During Choice." *Journal of Neuroscience* 29, no. 46 (2009): 14617–26.

Tansey, Katherine E., Keeley J. Brookes, Matthew J. Hill, Lynne E. Cochrane, Michael Gill, David Skuse, Catarina Correia, Astrid Vicente, Lindsey Kent, Louise

Gallagher, and Richard J. L. Anney. "Oxytocin Receptor (Oxtr) Does Not Play a Major Role in the Aetiology of Autism: Genetic and Molecular Studies." *Neuroscience Letters* 474, no. 3 (2010): 163–67.

Taylor, S. E., L. C. Klein, B. P. Lewis, T. L. Gruenewald, R. A. Gurung, and J. A. Updegraff. "Biobehavioral Responses to Stress in Females: Tend-and-Befriend, Not Fight-or-Flight." *Psychological Review* 107, no. 3 (2000): 411–29.

Tennie, Claudio, Josep Call, and Michael Tomasello. "Ratcheting up the Ratchet: On the Evolution of Cumulative Culture." *Philosophical Transactions of the Royal Society B: Biological Sciences* 364, no. 1528 (2009): 2405–15.

Thagard, Paul, and Karsten Verbeurgt. "Coherence as Constraint Satisfaction." *Cognitive Science* 22, no. 1: 1–24.

Thompson, R. R., K. George, J. C. Walton, S. P. Orr, and J. Benson. "Sex-Specific Influences of Vasopressin on Human Social Communication." *Proceedings of the National Academy of Sciences* 103, no. 20 (2006): 7889–94.

Thompson, William Forde. *Music, Thought, and Feeling: Understanding the Psychology of Music*. New York: Oxford University Press, 2009.

Tomasello, Michael. *The Cultural Origins of Human Cognition*. Cambridge, MA: Harvard University Press, 1999.

Tomasello, Michael, Malinda Carpenter, Josep Call, Tanya Behne, and Henrike Moll. "Understanding and Sharing Intentions: The Origins of Cultural Cognition." *Behavioral and Brain Sciences* 28, no. 5 (2005): 675–91.

Tooby, John, and Leda Cosmides, "The Psychological Foundations of Culture." In *The Adapted Mind: Evolutionary Psychology and the Generation of Culture*, edited by J. Barkow, L. Cosmides, and J. Tooby. New York: Oxford University Press, 1992.

Tost, Heike, Bhaskar Kolachana, Shabnam Hakimi, Herve Lemaitre, Beth A. Verchinski, Venkata S. Mattay, Daniel R. Weinberger, and Andreas Meyer-Lindenberg. "A Common Allele in the Oxytocin Receptor Gene (OXTR) Impacts Prosocial Temperament and Human Hypothalamic-Limbic Structure and Function." *Proceedings of the National Academy of Sciences* 107, no. 31 (2010): 13936–41.

Trivers, Robert L. "The Evolution of Reciprocal Altruism." *Quarterly Review of Biology* 46, no. 1 (1971): 35.

Tucker, Don M., Phan Luu, and Douglas Derryberry. "Love Hurts: The Evolution of Empathic Concern through the Encephalization of Nociceptive Capacity." *Development and Psychopathology* 17, no. 3 (2005): 699–713.

Turella, Luca, Andrea C. Pierno, Federico Tubaldi, and Umberto Castiello. "Mirror Neurons in Humans: Consisting or Confounding Evidence?" *Brain and Language* 108, no. 1 (2009): 10–21.

Turner, Leslie M., Adrian R. Young, Holger Rompler, Torsten Schoneberg, Steven M. Phelps, and Hopi E. Hoekstra. "Monogamy Evolves through Multiple Mechanisms: Evidence from V1ar in Deer Mice." *Molecular Biology and Evolution* 27, no. 6 (2010): 1269–78.

Uhlmann, Eric L., David A. Pizarro, David Tannenbaum, and Peter H. Ditto. "The Motivated Use of Moral Principles." *Judgment and Decision Making* 4 (2009): 476–91.

Valenstein, Elliot S. *Great and Desperate Cures: The Rise and Decline of Psychosurgery and Other Radical Treatments for Mental Illness*. New York: Basic Books, 1986.

Vasey, Natalie. "The Breeding System of Wild Red Ruffed Lemurs (*Varecia rubra*): A Preliminary Report." *Primates* 48, no. 1 (2007): 41–54.

Vigilant, L., M. Stoneking, H. Harpending, K. Hawkes, and A. C. Wilson. "African Populations and the Evolution of Human Mitochondrial DNA." *Science* 253, no. 5027 (1991): 1503–7.

Wallace, Edward C. "Put Vendors in Their Place." *New York Times*, April 17, 2010.

Walum, Hasse, Lars Westberg, Susanne Henningsson, Jenae M. Neiderhiser, David Reiss, Wilmar Igl, Jody M. Ganiban, Erica L. Spotts, Nancy L. Pedersen, Elias Eriksson, and Paul Lichtenstein. "Genetic Variation in the Vasopressin Receptor 1a Gene (*AVPR1A*) Associates with Pair-Bonding Behavior in Humans." *Proceedings of the National Academy of Sciences* 105, no. 37 (2008): 14153–56.

Wang, Zuoxin, Diane Toloczko, Larry J. Young, Kathleen Moody, John D. Newman, and Thomas R. Insel. "Vasopressin in the Forebrain of Common Marmosets (*Callithrix jacchus*): Studies with in Situ Hybridization, Immunocytochemistry and Receptor Autoradiography." *Brain Research* 768, no. 1–2 (1997): 147–56.

West, S. A., C. El Mouden, and A. Gardner. "16 Common Misconceptions about the Evolution of Cooperation in Humans." *Evolution and Human Behavior* (in press). http://www.zoo.ox.ac.uk/group/west/pubs.html.

Whiten, Andrew, Victoria Horner, and Frans B. M. de Waal. "Conformity to Cultural Norms of Tool Use in Chimpanzees." *Nature* 437, no. 7059 (2005): 737–40.

Whiten, Andrew, Antoine Spiteri, Victoria Horner, Kristin E. Bonnie, Susan P. Lambeth, Steven J Schapiro, and Frans B. M. de Waal. "Transmission of Multiple Traditions within and between Chimpanzee Groups." *Current Biology* 17, no. 12 (2007): 1038–43.

Wicker, Bruno, Christian Keysers, Jane Plailly, Jean-Pierre Royet, Vittorio Gallese, and Giacomo Rizzolatti. "Both of Us Disgusted in *My* Insula: The Common Neural Basis of Seeing and Feeling Disgust." *Neuron* 40, no. 3 (2003): 655–64.

Wild, Barbara, Michael Erb, Michael Eyb, Mathias Bartels, and Wolfgang Grodd. "Why Are Smiles Contagious? An fMRI Study of the Interaction between Perception of Facial Affect and Facial Movements." *Psychiatry Research* 123, no. 1 (2003): 17–36.

Williams, Justin, Andrew Whiten, and Tulika Singh. "A Systematic Review of Action Imitation in Autistic Spectrum Disorder." *Journal of Autism and Developmental Disorders* 34, no. 3 (2004): 285–99.

Williams-Gray, Caroline H., Adam Hampshire, Trevor W. Robbins, Adrian M. Owen, and Roger A. Barker. "Catechol O-Methyltransferase Val158met Genotype Influences Frontoparietal Activity During Planning in Patients with Parkinson's Disease." *Journal of Neuroscience* 27, no. 18 (2007): 4832–38.

Wilson, Catherine. "The Biological Basis and Ideational Superstructure of Ethics." *Canadian Journal of Philosophy* 26 (supplement) (2002): 211–44.

Winder-Rhodes, S. E., S.R. Chamberlain, M. I. Idris, T. W. Robbins, B. J. Sahakian, and U. Müller. "Effects of Modafinil and Prazosin on Cognitive and Physiological Functions in Healthy Volunteers." *Journal of Psychopharmacology* (in press).

Wood, Bernard A. *Human Evolution: A Very Short Introduction*. Oxford: Oxford University Press, 2005.

Woodward, James. "Interventionist Theories of Causation in Psychological Perspective." In *Causal Learning: Psychology, Philosophy and Computation* ed. A. Gopnik and L. Schulz, 19–36. New York: Oxford University Press, 2007.

Woodward, James, and John Allman. "Moral Intuition: Its Neural Substrates and Normative Significance." *Journal of Physiology–Paris* 101, no. 4–6 (2007): 179–202.

Wrangham, Richard W. "Ecology and Social Relationships in Two Species of Chimpanzees." In *Ecological Aspects of Social Evolution*, edited by D. Rubenstein and R. Wrangham, 352–78. Princeton, NJ: Princeton University Press, 1986.

Wrangham, Richard W., and Dale Peterson. *Demonic Males: Apes and the Origins of Human Violence*. Boston: Houghton Mifflin, 1996.

Young, Liane, and Rebecca Saxe. "An fMRI Investigation of Spontaneous Mental State Inference for Moral Judgment." *Journal of Cognitive Neuroscience* 21, no. 7 (2008): 1396–405.

Zak, P. J., A. A. Stanton, and S. Ahmadi. "Oxytocin Increases Generosity in Humans." *PLoS ONE* 2, no. 11 (2007): e1128.

Zald, David H., and Scott L. Rauch. *The Orbitofrontal Cortex*. New York: Oxford University Press, 2006.

Zhang, Ming, and Jing-Xia Cai. "Neonatal Tactile Stimulation Enhances Spatial Working Memory, Prefrontal Long-Term Potentiation, and D1 Receptor Activation in Adult Rats." *Neurobiology of Learning and Memory* 89, no. 4 (2008): 397–406.

Zimbardo, Philip G. *The Lucifer Effect: Understanding How Good People Turn Evil*. New York: Random House, 2007.

Acknowledgments

So many patient and smart scientists and philosophers have helped to teach me what they know. In particular, I wish to thank Roger Bingham, Simon Blackburn, Don Brown, Sue Carter, Bud Craig, Antonio Damasio, Hanna Damasio, Owen Flanagan, A. C. Grayling, Greg Hickok, Sarah Hrdy, Barry Keverne, George Koob, Randy Nesse, Jaak Panksepp, Don Pfaff, V. S. Ramachandran, Matt Ridley, Terry Sejnowski, Michael Stack, Ajit Varki, and Piotr Winkielman. Lt. Col. (USAF) Bill Casebeer, when studying at University California–San Diego, helped convince me that the stock arguments against a scientific account of the roots of morality were flawed, and that both Aristotle and Hume were moral philosophers for whom a neurobiology of morality would have made good sense. Ralph Greenspan and I jointly taught a graduate course on neurobiology and morality, an endeavor of great fun and enlightenment for me, and Ralph was instrumental in firming up ideas for this book. Additionally, I especially wish to thank Chris Suhler, a graduate student at UCSD, who has worked through many of the arguments and ideas in this book with me, and provided wisdom, wordsmithing, and good sense well beyond his years. Edwin McAmis is owed a special thanks for gracious support and for reading the manuscript with a lawyerly eye unmatched in its demands for clarity and coherence. Gratitude also goes to Sue Fellows, a philosopher, artist, and exacting critic. Mark Churchland and Anne Churchland, woodshedding critics both, helped me avoid assorted dumb mistakes and injected some new ways of thinking about the neurobiology of morality. Paul Churchland has worked through every thought with me, for nigh on forty-five years; I am never very clear about whether an idea is his or mine, and we agree it does not matter. Special thanks also to Senior Editor Rob Tempio at Princeton University Press, to copyeditor Jodi Beder, who in countless ways helped me ready the manuscript, and to Debbie Tegarden for keeping the wagons moving.

Index